LIVE LONGER NOW—

*important new discoveries in man's
continual quest to extend his life span*

The 2100 Program is the end product of many years of work by members of the Longevity Foundation of America. The Foundation is composed of professionals representing numerous areas of scientific research, many of whom joined together to create this book and the 2100 Program. You are not seeing just the views of the physician, but also the views of the organic chemist, the nutritionist, the biologist. It is a program combining multiviews drawn from many disciplines and from the results of many researchers throughout the world.

**A breakthrough book in hardcover—
now "must" reading in paperback!**

Berkley books by Nathan Pritikin

LIVE LONGER NOW (with Jon N. Leonard and Jack L. Hofer)

THE OFFICIAL PRITIKIN GUIDE TO RESTAURANT EATING
(with Ilene Pritikin)

Most Berkley Books are available at special quantity discounts for bulk purchases for sales promotions, premiums, fund raising, or educational use. Special books or book excerpts can also be created to fit specific needs.

For details, write or telephone Special Sales Markets, The Berkley Publishing Group, 200 Madison Avenue, New York, New York 10016; (212) 686-9820.

LIVE LONGER NOW:

The first one hundred years of your life: the 2100 program

BY JON N. LEONARD
JACK L. HOFER AND
NATHAN PRITIKIN

BERKLEY BOOKS, NEW YORK

LIVE LONGER NOW

A Berkley Book / published by arrangement with
the author

PRINTING HISTORY
Charter edition/ June 1978
Berkley edition / January 1986
Second printing / May 1986

All rights reserved.
Copyright © 1974 by Jon N. Leonard.
This book may not be reproduced in whole or in part,
by mimeograph or any other means, without permission.
For information address: The Berkley Publishing Group,
200 Madison Avenue, New York, NY 10016.

ISBN: 0-425-08691-7

A BERKLEY BOOK ® TM 757,375
Berkley Books are published by The Berkley Publishing Group,
200 Madison Avenue, New York, NY 10016.
The name "BERKLEY" and the stylized "B" with design
are trademarks belonging to Berkley Publishing Corporation.

PRINTED IN THE UNITED STATES OF AMERICA

Publisher's Foreword

This new and important book offers a fascinating concept for increasing your life-span. While the Longevity Foundation points out very clearly that their theory has not yet been tested on vast groups of people, the medical literature now available, they believe, strongly supports their concepts.

If, however, one is under treatment for some ailment, it is best to consult one's physician before entering upon the 2100 Program.

Acknowledgments

This book is based largely on writing and research done by men and women throughout the world in the various fields of nutrition, physical fitness, and degenerative diseases. So many direct or indirect sources have been used in the writing of this book that it would be impractical to acknowledge them all by name. Nevertheless, it is with a deep and humble sincerity that we acknowledge the vital contribution that many dedicated men and women have made to this book through their scientific and medical research.

The authors would also like to express their appreciation to the members of the Longevity Foundation of America who were involved in the research upon which this book is based, or in foundation activities related to the book's subject matter. For their invaluable contributions on all fronts, we thank them. Thanks are also due Robert Pritikin, who contributed toward the preparation of the chapter on exercise physiology, and Zelda Fields who helped compile the recipes.

A great debt of appreciation is owed to the many persons who have helped in the final stages of manuscript preparation. We wish to single out for special thanks Peggy Kuhn, Lynne MacInnis, Anne Serpa, Judy Ulstad, Bonnie Neelio, Linda Lee, and Myrna Levine for their assistance with typing, editing, preliminary artwork and critical review.

Finally, a note of gratitude is due those in our personal lives for their never-failing interest, encouragement and patience in this project.

Contents

NOTE: Read Part II first for a quick overview of the book.

Foreword v

Introduction ix

PART I · DEGENERATIVE DISEASES
What they are and how they are caused

1

CHAPTER 1: *A Massive Health Problem in the United States* — 3

CHAPTER 2: *How to Solve the Problem* — 17

CHAPTER 3: *The Role of Exercise* — 77

CHAPTER 4: *The Role of Nutrients: Vitamins, 85
Amino Acids, Minerals,
Carbohydrates, and Fats*

CHAPTER 5: *Other Players in the Game of Health* 116

PART II · GUIDE TO GOOD HEALTH 133

CHAPTER 6: *Longer Healthier Living* 135

CHAPTER 7: *The 2100 Food Program* 140

CHAPTER 8: *The 2100 Exercise Program* 178

CHAPTER 9: *Helpful Hints* 199

Appendix 210

Source Notes 219

Index 227

Introduction

This book speaks about fundamentally important human issues. It speaks about human nutrition and about human physical conditioning. It speaks also about well-known diseases * that may result if nutrition and physical conditioning are faulty. The book goes further, and recommends a program (the *2100 Program*) for eating and exercise that is designed to prevent and reverse these diseases. In fact this book goes so far as to say that if this recommended program were followed on a broad scale in this nation, then a dramatic improvement in national health and in the national average life span would result.

Indeed this book makes many strong assertions in an arena that is clearly of great importance to people. Therefore, it behooves us to spend some time examining where the conclusions in this book came from.

---

* Heart disease, diabetes, gout, arterial hypertension, atherosclerosis and cerebrovascular disease.

Introduction x

The results in this book are based primarily on an analysis of scientific literature. The literature analyzed is the international scientific literature on the subject of degenerative diseases. This literature consists of a great many journal articles and books, reporting the findings of literally hundreds of scientific studies that have been undertaken in the last forty or so years. Some of these studies investigated these diseases from the microscopic viewpoint of what happens to the body when they occur. Some of them investigated the disease from the viewpoint of which societies get them and which societies are free of them. Some of them investigated these diseases from the viewpoint of their possible patterns of genetic transmission. Still other studies investigated them from the subtle viewpoint of the degree to which they are mere artifacts of our ever-changing ability to detect them. All of these various kinds of studies were part of the literature that was analyzed in drawing the results for this book.

The literature analysis was done by the Longevity Foundation of America. The Longevity Foundation is a small research institute[*] with a multidisciplinary staff. Thus in analyzing the literature, a multidisciplinary approach was taken. Involved in the analysis were people from many disciplines other than the discipline of medicine. Physics, chemistry, psychology, computer science, mathematical logic, and engineering are some of the disciplines that were involved in the analysis of the literature.

This book is a result of applying a multidisciplinary staff to the literature already in existence regarding degenerative diseases. No new experiments were carried out by the Foundation; not a test tube was lifted. Yet conclusions that were reached are novel, and of tremendous importance.

At this point one might reasonably ask: "If these conclu-

---

[*] The Foundation has fourteen members, who do the work of the Foundation, and foot the Foundation's bills.

sions are correct, then why didn't some group other than the Longevity Foundation arrive at them first? After all, these conclusions must obviously have lain hidden in the data already gathered. Why weren't they spotted by some larger and more powerful research group some time ago?"

As it happens, many of the pieces that make up the conclusions of this book *were* discovered by other researchers first. So in some sense the intuitive feeling that the big research institutes should have seen things first is correct. But the whole picture as we have drawn it here, has not been perceived before. Pieces of it were seen, but in isolation from each other. The broad relationships among these pieces remained hidden.

The question still remains: "Why did other larger institutions not see this big picture first?" Perhaps the reason lies in the use of the multidisciplinary team of scientists. Most research teams, particularly in the study of disease, consist of a relatively narrow set of scientific disciplines. This narrowness, while possibly a good thing for the pursuit of penetrating studies in a narrow specialty, may nevertheless be a counter-productive thing for seeing the big picture.

Perhaps the reason lies in some direction other than the makeup of the research team. In any case, the conclusions drawn by the Foundation are sweepingly different than those drawn by others.

Are the conclusions of this book good ones? If logic and reason are good tools for discovering the secrets of nature, then they are. In deciding what is true about the natural universe, science really has only one tool. That tool is the comparison of a theory about nature with the findings that exist concerning what happens in nature. When the theory is consistent with all of the known facts, and when it can accurately predict other facts, it is accepted as fact itself. It becomes a law of nature.

What we discuss in this book is really a theory about

nature; a theory about how nutrition and physical exertion relate to degenerative diseases. The theory discussed here was found to have the following properties. It was found to be consistent with the known facts concerning nutrition, exertion, and degenerative disease. It was found to accurately predict natural phenomena concerning nutrition, exertion, and degenerative disease. No other existing theory was found to have those properties. Nor could the Foundation create a different one meeting the requirements of consistency with known facts and predictive powers. Thus the theory about nature that is presented in this book is as close to a fact about nature as can be generated at this time. Not only is it as good a picture of nature as we can get; the recommendations it implies are safe. Thus the program recommended here has no potential for harm, yet it has tremendous potential for good.

This book is written for the layman. Not every conclusion is documented by supporting theoretical arguments. Such a technical rationale might be interesting to the expert, but it might also jeopardize the usefulness of this book to the layman. Therefore, rationale and reference to the literature is presented only on particularly controversial points.

Do the Recommendations in This Book Work in Practice?

The recommendations in this book are embodied in the *2100 Program* described in Part II. Will the 2100 Program work in practice? The authors of this book believe that it will. The evidence in the international literature is overwhelmingly in support of it. But many people would argue that to know for certain whether or not the 2100 Program would dramatically improve health and longevity in this country, the Program would have to be actually tested first on millions of people here. Such a test has of course not been made on the 2100 Program. Nor is such a test likely to be made. Nevertheless, people within and outside the Foundation have adopted the 2100 Program with phenomenal results.

Everyone who has adopted the 2100 Program, whether healthy or not, has been able to exert dramatic control over the blood components that normally indicate a potential for, or a presence of, degenerative diseases. For example, triglyceride levels and cholesterol levels in the blood can easily be reduced to startlingly low levels via the 2100 Program, and every person who has adopted the Program has experienced this.

In addition, those people who have begun the 2100 Program while in the throes of one or more of the degenerative diseases have shown remarkable reversal of their condition. Examples of these reversals are provided below. In each of these seven examples, the person involved adopted the 2100 Program for the duration indicated. If rigorous adherence was kept to the 2100 Program diet (as the diet is defined in Part II), then it is estimated that the following daily dietary intakes apply:

Fat	5 to 10% of daily calories (⅛ to ¼ of American average)
Sugar, honey, etc.	0 grams (American average is greater than 100 grams per day)
Salt	1 to 2 grams (about ⅒ of American average)
Caffeine	5 to 10 mg. (American average greater than 400 mg.)
Cholesterol	less than 100 mg. (about ⅛ of American average)

If rigorous adherence was kept to the 2100 Program exercise regimen (as the regimen is defined in Part II), then three to four hours of endurance activities were undertaken weekly.

Example 1 (J.S. and E.W.)

J.S. and E.W. are both great-grandmothers now in their eighties. Three years ago J.S. was being treated for high blood pressure and angina,* and was taking medication for both. At that time circulation was so poor in her legs that she could not walk 100 yards without having to stop because of leg pains.

At the same time E.W. was in even worse shape. She too required medication for hypertension and angina, and she too had the circulatory symptoms of atherosclerosis: leg pains upon walking, and cold extremities in all weather. E.W. was afraid to leave her house for fear that if she had to sit down to rest or if she fell down, she would not be able to get up again. In fact, she could not walk 50 feet without literally having to be carried back home.

Concerned relatives introduced these two ladies to a joint 2100 diet/exercise program three years ago. For these laides, their "endurance activities" at first amounted to only walks around their living rooms. Their diets were immediately altered to the 2100 Program of very low fats, cholesterol, salt, caffeine, and sugar. Within a matter of six weeks endurance activities for both ladies had expanded to outdoor walking, and within twenty-four months both ladies were off all medications and are still off at this time.

Today J.S. walks a mile daily, jogs a half mile, rides the stationary bicycle six miles, lifts weights twice a week and swims regularly. E.W. accompanies J.S. in her activities, except that E.W. jogs one and one quarter miles, and rides the stationary bicycle 15 miles per day. They are both still adhering to the 2100 Diet Program.

---

* Angina is an excruciating viselike pain in the chest due to coronary insufficiency. People who have had it often say that it is the worst pain they have ever experienced.

Example 2 (R.D.)

R.D. was diagnosed as a diabetic when she was three years old, at which time she was started on daily insulin injections. By the time she was 19 years old, her diabetes was severe. She was taking 60 units of insulin every day, was swollen with edema, was having difficulty avoiding diabetic coma on the one hand, and insulin shock on the other, and was fearful of blindness from diabetic retinopathy.

R.D. started on a rigid 2100 Program at the beginning of the summer vacation, at age 19. By the end of six weeks she had kept successful adherence to the 2100 Program low fat, zero sugar diet, and was jogging two miles each day. By that time she had lost the swelling of edema and twenty pounds of weight, mostly fluid. By the end of the summer vacation, she had worked her way down to a mere six units of insulin per day (under her doctor's daily supervision, an absence of glucose and ketones from the urine being the criterion used for reducing the insulin by one or two units). This was less than her insulin intake had been since she was a very small child.

Example 3 (J.G.)

J.G. had been taking drugs for 10 years for high blood pressure. Even with drugs his blood pressure never got below 160/90 the entire ten-year time span, and at times was much higher. One year ago J.G., then age 62, decided to try the 2100 Program. Within three months of starting the program he was able to stop taking all high blood pressure medication. Today he remains completely free of antihypertensive drugs, is still on the 2100 Program, and has a blood pressure of 127/83.

Example 4 (M.T.)

M.T. had been having painful and crippling attacks of gout in his great toes. After his last attack one year ago at age

51, he made the decision to begin the 2100 Program. Within weeks his toes were completely normal, he has had no symptoms since, and he is still on the 2100 Program.

Example 5 (R.P.)

R.P. was diagnosed as diabetic ten years ago. He had been taking oral medication for diabetes ever since his diagnosis. Two years ago at age 52, concerned with blindness from diabetic retinopathy and facing other complications of diabetes, R.P. decided to try the 2100 Program. Today R.P. takes no drugs whatever, and all clinical evidence of diabetes has disappeared. He runs one and one half miles each day, and is still on the 2100 Program Diet regimen.

Example 6 (N.I.)

Several years ago at age 48, N.I. was diagnosed as having a severe case of coronary insufficiency, based on EKG studies made by his cardiologist. At that time he was advised to abandon all exercise other than short, slow walks. His cholesterol level then was over 300 mg.%. Fearful of an imminent heart attack, yet not wishing to remain a semi-invalid, N.I. decided to try the 2100 Program. He switched to the 2100 Program diet and began a cardiovascular conditioning program through slow and careful endurance activities per the 2100 Exercise Program.

Today, two years later he is still on the very low fat, low cholesterol regimen of the 2100 Program Diet. His cholesterol level has dropped to the remarkably low level of 125 mg.%. He is also still on the 2100 Exercise Program: N.I. is now running five miles four times a week.

About This Book

This book is about living. It is a book that tells how to live to an old age, and how to avoid the pitfalls of heart disease, diabetes, senility and other degenerative diseases along the way. If you are healthy now, and want to live a long, active

life, this is a book for you. It will tell you about staying healthy by avoiding the calamity of degenerative diseases.*
If you are not healthy now and are suffering from any number of ailments of the degenerative type, then this is a book for you as well. It will show you where you went wrong, and how to get back on the right track and stay there.

The book is divided into two parts. Part I tells the story of degenerative diseases, where they come from and what they do to us, while Part II tells you what you have to do to prevent and reverse degenerative diseases. Part II is a simple How-to-Do-It guide to good health, and will be an invaluable tool in getting yourself into the mainstream of good health. If you want to get a quick start on a health program for yourself, you can go directly to Part II and skip over Part I altogether. If you want to learn about what degenerative diseases are and how they work their harm in the body, however, you need to read Part I as well.

A subtitle of the book is the 2100 Program. This subtitle was chosen because the eating/exercise program in this book will help you live as long as a person born in the year 2100 would live. People who watch life-span trends tell us that the average life span probably won't hit 90 years until sometime after the year 2100. But for you personally this does not have to be the case. You can immeasurably increase your chances of having a 2100 life span by applying the eating and exercise principles laid out in the book.

About Living a Long Time

Perhaps you feel that reaching the age of 90 is something that you shouldn't worry about at your present age. In case you do feel this way, there are some things you should know. You should know that the way you eat and the way you

---

* Degenerative diseases refers to heart disease, diabetes, atherosclerosis, arterial hypertension, cerebrovascular disease, and gout.

exercise today may strongly affect how pleasant or unpleasant your life will be in the years from about 50 onward. By not thinking about your future now you may do a great deal more to yourself than merely shorten your life span by 20 years or so. You may be condemning yourself to a painful and extended period of decrepitude and illness, beginning somewhere in your fifties and growing in severity until your death. You cannot start too young to prevent this situation: the younger the better.

If you follow the 2100 Program recommendations on eating and exercise your chances of being able to stand at age 50 and look forward to many healthy years of activity and productivity will be greatly increased. Perhaps equally as important, you are much more likely to be an asset to your family and to society rather than a liability in your later years.

About the Quality of Life

Most of us get a certain kind of pleasure from thinking about ourselves living to a healthy and happy ripe old age of 90. But we need also to think about how the quality of life in the nation would be affected if we were all to achieve this goal. It might, for instance, be thought that living a long lifetime would somehow place a drain on society's young people. Since we tend to think of 90-year-olds as Medicare cases, we can easily see ourselves as having to pay more taxes to support an ever-growing group of old people—people who are taking up space in a crowded world that might very well be better utilized by younger blood. However, there are better ways to look at what would happen.

In the first place, the 2100 Program has the effect of extending the middle years, not the old ones. This means that you may live 20 years longer, but your age 65 would be more like age 45, and age 90 would be more like age 70. Extra middle years give you more years while your productivity is high, causing your net worth to society to go up. If we assume that a man's most productive time today amounts to only about 30 years (perhaps it's really more than that), then an extra 20 years of high productivity increases his lifetime output by 67 percent.

In the second place, in today's world by the time a man has raised his family, he has usually passed the prime of his life. The obstacles that stand in the way of his changing the course of his life at that time are often very great. Most of the obstacles crop up because the time he has left to live is limited. Since his healthy years are numbered, it is easy for him to think that the best thing for him to do is just "get along" until his time to die comes. With 20 years of full prime life still ahead of him, however, these obstacles could be overcome, and new careers could be started. Those extra middle years would provide more opportunities, as well as more productivity for the members of our society.

Of course productivity and opportunity are not the whole answer to the question of the quality of life. There is the problem of overpopulation and the question of what effect a longer lifetime will have on that problem. It has been shown [98] that long lifetimes have a very small effect on the population's growth, when compared with other population pressures such as the birth rate. Here in the United States, for example, the increase in population caused by a *permanent* increase in the average lifespan from 70 to 90 is more than offset by a reduction of the average multichild family from four to three children *for only one generation*.[98] Thus the population pressure generated by long lifetimes is comparatively small.

About the 2100 Program

The 2100 Program is the end product of many man years of work by members of the Longevity Foundation of America. The Foundation is composed of professionals representing numerous areas of scientific research, many of whom joined together to create this book and the 2100 Program. To you this means that you are seeing all sides of the picture in the 2100 Program. You are not seeing just the views of the physician, but also the views of the organic chemist, the nutritionist, and the biologist. Your 2100 Program is not just a nutritionist's idea of how to live a long healthy life anymore than it is simply a physician's or chemist's. It is a program combining multiviews drawn from many disciplines and the results of many researchers throughout the world.

It is no longer a mystery why heart disease, diabetes, and the other degenerative diseases have increased so much in the past 50 years. The facts are in. But it takes stepping back and getting a perspective on a lot of data all at once. The Longevity Foundation took that step back and looked at the mountains of research results that currently exist. The solution to the degenerative disease puzzle lay there among the facts like a pearl among pebbles. The solution might not have been there, or it might have been too obscure to be seen. But it was there, and it was seen; furthermore, it turned out to be a very simple one indeed: A matter of what we have been eating and doing with our bodies. In the next few chapters we will lay out, in the 2100 Program, the facts of the solution and how to use it.

DEGENERATIVE DISEASES

/ PART 1

*What they are
and how they are caused*

CHAPTER 1

A Massive Health Problem in the United States

Changing Patterns of Disease

In 1910 tuberculosis (TB) was the single largest cause of death in the United States.[1] It accounted for more than 100,000 annual deaths and untold suffering and misery. TB was commonly called "consumption," because the disease seemed to consume the flesh and vitality of its victim and left behind only a shadow of the person it victimized. It is difficult to appreciate today how bad things were then. In 1910 TB sanatoriums were scattered all over the country. The disease victims would go to these sanatoriums to avail themselves of the special treatments and therapies that might be offered. Cures were rare and quackery abounded, however, and more often than not a TB sanatorium was a place where one went to die.

But things have changed since 1910. Today, although tuberculosis still causes a few deaths each year, we can confidently say that it is a conquered disease. The number of people who will die of TB this year will be less than 1 percent of the number who died in 1910, just as it has been less than 1 percent every year for the last several years. The sanatoriums have nearly all closed their doors. With several potent antibiotic drugs that are effective against TB, the medical profession can quickly bring about a cure in almost every instance of this disease.

Thus TB, once the greatest of the infective diseases, has been overcome. Not only has TB been overcome, but also most of the infective diseases that plagued Americans early in this century have been virtually defeated. Outbreaks of typhoid fever, malaria, and smallpox killed many thousands in 1910. Scarlet fever, whooping cough and measles killed even more the same year. Today all these infective diseases have practically disappeared as causes of death in the United States.

This is very good. We can be justifiably proud of such a major medical achievement in just a few generations. But should we be satisfied with the state of health in the United States today, now that such marvelous advances have come about? The answer is *no*, we should not be satisfied. No one in the medical profession is satisfied with the current state of health of the majority of Americans. The reason is that even though we have conquered infective diseases, we have not made the least dent in another class of diseases, the degenerative diseases.

As we have already mentioned, the degenerative diseases discussed here are: heart disease, atherosclerosis, cerebrovascular disease (stroke), diabetes, arterial hypertension, and gout. These diseases are called degenerative diseases because they each involve the degenerative breakdown of millions of different body cells. "Degenerative diseases" is an apt description of these diseases for another reason, too. Not only do they involve the degenerative breakdown of individual body cells, they involve the degenerative breakdown of the whole person as well. A person, in extreme cases, might begin with a case of diabetes and soon find himself with a fullblown case of hardened arteries. The same person might then experience a heart attack, develop high blood pressure, and finally suffer a stroke. The point is that a person with a degenerative disease will often experience massive degeneration of his entire body over a period of time. Thus degenerative diseases are aptly named.

Although TB killed more people in 1910 than any other disease, heart disease, the major degenerative disease, came in a close second.[1] Since 1910 we have made little progress in the prevention of heart disease in this country. Nearly six times as many people will die of heart disease this year as died in 1910. Actually things are not six times as bad now as they were in 1910. After all, other things being equal, one would expect more Americans to die of heart disease today than in 1910 because there are a lot more people in the United States today than there were in 1910. In addition, today there are a lot more people in the older age brackets where heart disease strikes hardest.

Taking all complicating factors into account, however, it can be shown that your chances of dying from heart disease today are very nearly what they were in 1910. This is true even though a tremendous medical technology has been developed to deal with heart problems. Even though the thoracic surgeon can perform heart transplants, implant artificial heart valves and supplement the heart's arteries with veins transplanted from the leg, nevertheless, the average American is about as likely to die this year of heart disease as he would have been in the year 1910.

The story with cerebrovascular disease is essentially the same as the story with heart disease. The average person appears to be about as likely to die of cerebrovascular disease today as he ever was,[99] despite the fact that deaths from cerebral hemorrhages have evidently declined significantly since the introduction of effective antihypertensive drugs [100] in 1956. Atherosclerosis, which as we shall see later is a precursor to both heart disease and cerebrovascular disease, also appears not to have abated over the years.

Fatalities from the other degenerative diseases—arterial hypertension, diabetes, and gout—are less likely to occur today than previously. However, the number of deaths from heart disease, cerebrovascular disease, and atherosclerosis is so much greater than the number of deaths from the other three degenerative diseases that our progress in degenerative diseases as a class is measured primarily by our progress with heart disease, cerebrovascular disease, and atherosclerosis alone.

Unfortunately, our progress with these three diseases is none too good. In fact, the major medical picture of the last 60 years is essentially this: We have stripped away nearly all of the infective causes of death, and what is left over is a core of degenerative diseases that we have not yet been able to crack.

Figure 1 on the facing page shows graphically how this core of degenerative diseases has been exposed after the infective diseases have been eroded away by medical progress. The figure shows changing death rates for people * in the 35- to 45-year-old age bracket between 1920 and 1967. Only the major degenerative disease, heart disease, is shown, but all the infective diseases are lumped together. Notice how the infective disease death rate dropped to

* The figure shows data for white males only. Because of inadequacies in the tabulation of census data in past years for blacks and for females, the only easy way to obtain comparable statistics for the entire United States over any significant period of time is to employ white males exclusively. It appears that similar charts for females and blacks would show similar effects, however.

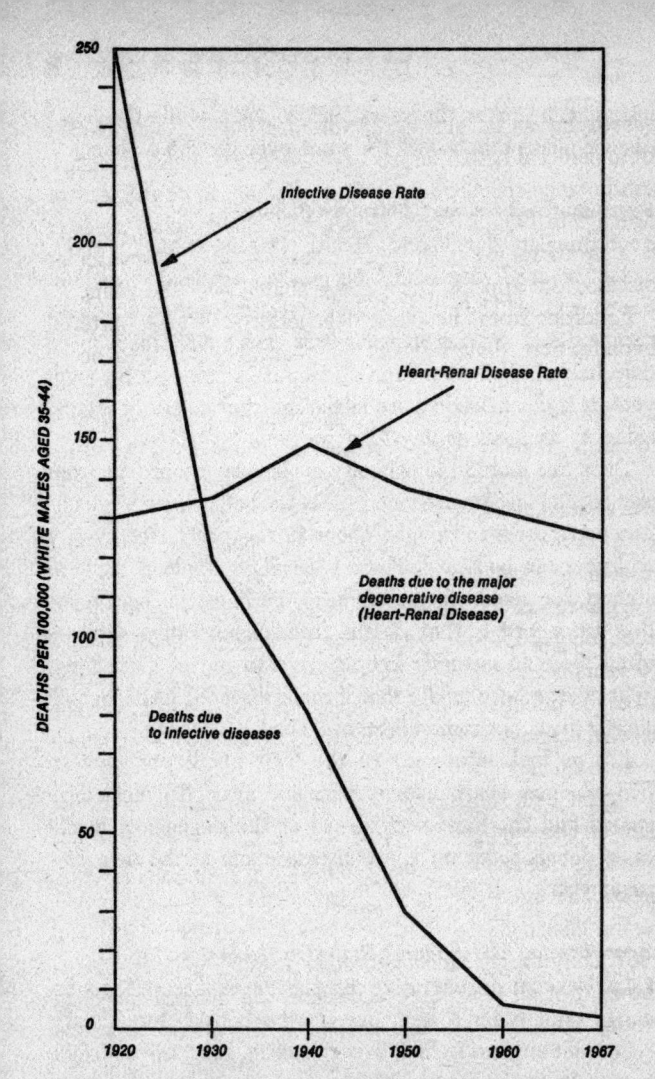

Figure 1. Deaths Due to Infective Diseases and the Major Degenerative Disease (Heart-Renal Disease) Between the Years 1920 and 1967 for People in the 35 to 44 Age Bracket.

insignificance over the years 1920 to 1967, while the heart disease death rate stayed the same over the same years.[1]

Degenerative Diseases: A Modern Plague

According to the World Health Organization (WHO), today we are living with "the greatest epidemic mankind has ever faced."[2] In the United States more than a million people die of degenerative diseases each year. This is more than half of all deaths from all causes in this country each year. It is clear that we are in the midst of a major medical calamity as great as anything we have ever faced.

Does this incredible calamity evoke any cry of fear from the people, any impassioned pleas for help, as such calamities have always brought about in the past? Not even a whimper can be heard. There is hardly a ripple of concern among the people in this country. Perhaps the reason for this unconcern is that deaths from degenerative diseases often seem so natural: People have to die of something. What better way to die than from a diseased heart, which simply gives out some night while one is sleeping.

Let us look into some of the facts about our modern plague. Since heart disease is far and away the most dangerous and the most widespread of the degenerative diseases, let us focus on heart disease alone in the next few paragraphs.

Heart Disease Starts Young in the United States

Like the other degenerative diseases, heart disease* is ordinarily present for a long time in the body before drastic symptoms appear. In fact, in our country, heart disease often begins in the early twenties, growing worse as the years pass until finally the inevitable heart attack strikes. For most

---

* In this section we will be talking about coronary artery disease, a form of atherosclerosis. However, we shall refer to it simply as heart disease, for ease of discussion.

people the first heart attack does not come until the fifties or sixties. But for thousands of people every year, the first heart attack comes in the twenties.[101] Occasionally even a person in his teens may experience a fatal heart attack.

It is a big surprise for most people to think of heart disease as being a part of the early twenties, but this is nevertheless evidently so. Several studies have been done to determine how widespread heart disease is in young people. Such studies have been difficult to do, however. The reason for this is that after a person has died it many times can be determined whether or not that person had a case of heart disease while he was living. But it has been relatively hard to know, while a person *is* living, whether or not that person has heart disease. Thus studies of how much heart disease is present in seemingly healthy young people are not easy to perform.

However, during the Korean and Vietnam wars, many young men were killed, who were in all ways healthy right up until the time they met death on the battlefield. In both of these wars a careful study was performed on the hearts of hundreds of young soldiers killed in battle to see how widespread heart disease was in American soldiers.

Before discussing the results of these wartime studies, we need to say a word about how we can tell that a heart is diseased. Almost all heart attacks are caused, indirectly, by the arteries that carry blood around in the body. In our country, people's arteries tend to develop plaques, which are like festering sores on the inside walls of the arteries. Plaques have a tendency to grow in size, and when they do, they can block off the flow of blood in various arteries in the body. If some of the arteries that deliver blood to the heart muscle (the coronary arteries) become blocked, then part of the heart muscle may die from lack of blood. When this happens to a person, he suffers a type of heart attack known as an *infarction*.

Infarctions are not the only type of heart attack that can occur. Another type is the *fibrillation,* wherein the heartbeat rhythm is disturbed so greatly that instead of pumping with strong coordinated contractions, the heart muscle trembles and jitters in an uncoordinated way. Like the infarction, the fibrillation is also caused by a blocking of some of the coronary arteries. The blockage in this case is the type resulting in an uneven supply of blood to different parts of the muscle, which in turn can lead to the uncoordinated heart contraction process that is characteristic of the fibrillation.

Even if the person has never had an actual heart attack, we can rate the amount of heart disease he has by the amount of plaque blockage that he has in the coronary arteries. This is exactly what was done with hundreds of young American soldiers who were killed in Korea and Vietnam. The amount of heart disease present in these young men was determined by careful autopsy examination of their arteries just after they met their death. In Korea, 300 autopsies were performed,[3] and in more than half of the cases, artery damage from plaques was obvious in the coronary arteries. The average age of the men at the time of their deaths was about 22 years. In 1971, more than 100 autopsies were performed on American soldiers killed in South Vietnam using more advanced methods of determining artery damage.[4] In this case it was found that 45 percent of the autopsies showed evidence of medium artery damage. In another 5 percent of the autopsies there was evidence of severe artery damage. The average age of the soldiers in the South Vietnam case was also about 22 years.

It is a safe bet that the young Americans killed in Korea and South Vietnam are just like the rest of the young men back home as far as heart disease is concerned. Therefore, the average American man of the same age is likely to have the same amount of heart disease as the group of men studied in Korea and Vietnam. This means that today about half of the American men in their early twenties have already started building up their case of heart disease. Data regarding the prevalence of heart disease in young women is harder to come by, and for this reason no one knows how prevalent heart disease is in young women.

United States Rates Poorly

Heart disease does not show up in the young men of every country. In Japan, young men have been autopsied in a way similar to the American war casualties, and it has been discovered that artery damage is almost absent. Not only does Japan have clean arteries in its young men, but in addition, heart disease in older Japanese is much lower than it is in older Americans.

An international study of heart disease in more than 12,000 middle-aged men from seven countries showed that the United States ranked second highest for heart disease while Japan rated lowest.[9] Heart disease in the 40- to 59-year-old age bracket is nearly nine times as common in the United States as in Japan.

Greece, Yugoslavia, Italy, and the Netherlands also rated lower than the United States for heart disease in the studied age bracket. Greece had only a fifth the U.S. rate of heart disease, while Yugoslavia had a rate of less than a third, and Italy about one half the rate of the U.S. The Netherlands had a heart disease rate which was about 30 percent less than the American heart disease rate. Only Finland had a higher heart disease rate than ours. Finland's rate was about 10 percent higher than the American rate.

Heart Disease Is Not a Matter of Weakening or a Fact of Age

The fact that heart disease is present in American youth, but not in the youth of some other countries, is very important. It is an important fact because it illustrates again that heart disease is an organic, growing disease like cancer or TB and not just a condition of getting old. It is tempting to believe that U.S. heart disease rates are high because some high percentage of "weaklings" are saved by the miraculous powers of American medical science (weaklings who then survive long enough to get heart disease in later life), whereas in other countries with lower medical standards, these same weaker individuals would die young of any number of ailments before they got old enough to reach the point at which heart disease could develop. If this were indeed true, then in fact the heart disease potential (namely, plaque-filled arteries) of the youth in any country would be about the same as for the youth in our country. Only time and exposure to disease would filter out the weaker individuals in other countries so as to produce the differences in heart disease rates that can be seen between this country and others. But the youth would be the same. The fact that the youth in other countries are not the same as those here, that, in fact, American youth—both the strong and the weak—have the beginnings of heart disease, while the strong and the weak youth in some other countries have no heart disease at all, is a very important fact indeed. This fact shows us that:

1. Heart disease is not a condition of age.
2. Heart disease is not an "artifact" produced by saving weak people.

Clean Bill of Health No Guarantee

It is clear that heart disease is a major American health problem that can potentially affect each of us. Unfortunately, the way things work right now, our medical system is neither able to prevent a given person from developing heart disease nor likely to inform any given person whether or not he even has heart disease until the disease has pro-

A Massive Health Problem in the United States 13

gressed to the dangerous stage. In fact, a person can go to his doctor, get a complete physical exam and get a clean bill of health, and yet die the next day of a heart attack.

Most of us have heard of people who were in seemingly perfect health but who died suddenly of a heart attack while shoveling snow, playing cards, or engaging in some other ordinary activity. There simply is not any widely used means to predict in advance that these people were in grave danger of dying from a heart attack.* An interesting case showing how true this is involved an apparently healthy USN fighter pilot who died suddenly of a heart attack.[5] On reviewing his health records, it was found that only three weeks before, he had finished an extensive battery of USN flight examinations designed to find even the slightest trace of any heart disease. The exams had not found anything significantly wrong with him, and he had been certified for flight status. Yet he was only three weeks away from his grave at the time the exams were completed.

A few months ago one of this book's authors was in the head offices of a large American corporation meeting with the company's founder. The founder is a health enthusiast who not only personally supports a nutrition research foundation but also has provided a very progressive medical program for all of the company's employees. All employees are periodically given medical examinations at company expense, and any determined medical problems are taken care of by company insurance policies.

The scheduled meeting with the founder never got off the ground. In the middle of the meeting a very agitated secretary broke in to say that one of the lobby guards just

---

* There are procedures (treadmill or angiograph) that can determine the existence of coronary artery disease in many cases. Unfortunately these procedures are not fully effective, nor are they in sufficiently wide use to benefit a majority of the population.

outside the door had been stricken by a heart attack. Within hours the guard died.

This particular guard had been with the corporation for many years and had acted over the years as a personal assistant to the founder himself. Needless to say this was a tragic event for everyone concerned. Even with the progressive medical programs provided for all employees, this heart attack was in no way foreseen.

Recently Lewis Kuller of Johns Hopkins University studied all deaths in a one-year time period for all people between ages 20 and 64 in the city of Baltimore.[6] Kuller found that even if he ignored traffic and other violent deaths, 32 percent of all the deaths in Baltimore in that year were sudden and unexpected, and most of these were caused by heart attacks. About half of the heart-attack victims had never had any sign of heart disease before they died. The first and last symptom they ever experienced was their fatal heart attack. About a fourth of all the people who suffered fatal heart attacks had just been to see their doctors within a week before their attacks.

It does not matter, therefore, if your doctor has just given you a clean bill of health—a heart attack may be just around the cornor. The picture in the United States is a pretty grim one. Heart disease has grown to epidemic proportions. Our medical system is not able to effectively detect impending heart attacks despite all of our medical technology. Heart attacks can strike anywhere, anytime, without warning.

Myth of U.S. Life Expectancies

We have just described some of the features of this country's number one health problem: heart disease. Despite the obvious magnitude of this health problem, there are always people who say: "No matter how much heart disease you say we have, things have got to be better now than

A Massive Health Problem in the United States 15

ever before, because my life expectancy is longer, and that's all that counts to me." In this last section, therefore, we will deal with the "myth of long-life expectancy."

For years we in the United States have been led to believe that we have the world's healthiest society. One reason that it is easy to believe this has to do with life-expectancy statistics. If you look at the life tables compiled by the U.S. Department of Health, Education, and Welfare (HEW), you find that a white male born today can "expect" to live to about age 67. What this means is that if the death rates in the country stay exactly as they are today throughout the lifetime of this baby boy, then *on the average* he will live to be 67. Some of the baby boys born today will thus die at 20, some will die at 100, but the average age of death will be 67. The important point here is that if a lot of babies die young, say because of birth complications or maybe because of childhood diseases such as measles or mumps, then this average age of death will drop down to a lot lower figure. So even if everybody were then to live on till he's 100, this expected length of life published by HEW could still be a very low number, due to a large number of childhood deaths.

As a matter of fact, a situation pretty much like this actually prevailed around the turn of the century here in America. At that time the expected length of life for a white male baby was only about 50 years. Today it is 67. That sounds impressive. It sounds as if people are living to be a lot older than they did in the past.

But this is false. The truth is: In the early 1900s *a baby was so likely to die in childhood of childhood diseases and complications* that the mathematical averages were brought way down, and the expected life span was therefore low. But once a person got past childhood he could expect to live nearly as long as a person today. In fact, in 1920 a white male 50 years of age could reasonably expect to live on to age 72.25. Today he can expect to live on to age 73. That is a difference of only about nine months even though generations of medical science and progress have happened between 1920 and now. Today we have penicillin, heart transplants and space age drugs, yet there is really little difference in how long a fully grown person can live today as compared to the early part of this century.

This situation underscores the fact that one cannot judge the health of adult Americans solely on the basis of life expectancy figures. This is the trap into which we nevertheless have fallen. We might take a look at Bolivia * for instance, and see that the expected length of life for a male baby is 49 years, 9 months. Since ours is so much longer (67+), we might think that Bolivians simply do not have very many old people; and we might also think that the few old people they have must indeed be sickly. But before we congratulate ourselves on how healthy we must be in this country compared to Bolivia, let us look at a different statistic. Instead of comparing ourselves with the Bolivian baby boy, let's compare ourselves with the 40-year-old Bolivian man. In Bolivia, a 40-year-old man can expect to live to 73 years, 5 months. On the other hand, in this country, a 40-year-old white male can expect to live only to 71 years, 5 months. That is two years less than the Bolivian. Given the fact that in America we have access to a health technology that far exceeds what is available to the Bolivian, this two-year difference is quite significant.

How should we rate our health then? Is our health situation really better than the Bolivians? Maybe, in some sense, it is for the newborn American baby, but it is certainly not better for the 40-year-old American man.

---

* These figures were compiled about 1950 in Bolivia.

CHAPTER 2

How to Solve the Problem

In the last chapter we discussed how big the degenerative disease problem is. Luckily for anyone who would like to stay healthy, a great deal can be done to prevent and reverse degenerative diseases with what we know right now. Prevention and reversal of these diseases can be approached without drugs or medical equipment of any kind. All that is needed is care in what one eats, and how one exercises one's body. It is as simple as that.

This situation is a lot different from the situation for infective diseases. Infective diseases of all kinds were conquered during the last 50 years largely because we were able to develop drugs to attack the infective agents. In fact, without drugs we would still be in real trouble from many of the infective diseases. But the same is not true of degenerative diseases. We do not have to wait for medical breakthroughs to treat them. Drugs are not needed and are not even desirable.

In this chapter we will talk about three degenerative diseases: atherosclerosis, diabetes, and arterial hypertension. We shall devote a section to each one. The understandings generated in the discussions of these degenerative diseases will enable us to formulate the principles necessary for the treatment and prevention of the other degenerative diseases as well.

Atherosclerosis * is a disease of the arteries which causes most kinds of heart disease and most kinds of stroke. If you prevent atherosclerosis you also prevent nearly every important kind of heart disease ** and stroke.

Diabetes is a disease in which the body cells lose much of their ability to burn sugar. When this happens sugar is not used properly in the body and as a result a diabetic person develops high levels of sugar in his blood and in his urine. Since the diabetic's body cells cannot burn sugar for energy, they have to use other sources in the body for energy in order to stay alive. Consequently, a diabetic person begins to use body fat and even body protein for fuel, creating by-products in the body that may cause diabetic coma or death.

Arterial hypertension, or simply hypertension, is a disease in which the blood pressure in the arteries rises to dangerously high levels. Hypertension appears to worsen the con-

---

* Atherosclerosis is sometimes confused with arteriosclerosis. Atherosclerosis refers to a specific disease condition, which we describe in some detail in this chapter. Arteriosclerosis, however, in its general usage, refers to the *class* of conditions that might be described as "pathological changes in the arteries." Thus atherosclerosis might be considered to be a type of arteriosclerosis. Arteriosclerosis is often used as a synonym for "hardening of the arteries." This is a more restricted usage of the word than the aforementioned general usage.

** Even though heart disease is the number one killer, we shall focus not on heart disease, but rather on atherosclerosis because of the crucial role atherosclerosis plays in causing other degenerative diseases. Heart disease and atherosclerosis are closely related and in the ensuing pages our discussion of atherosclerosis also relies heavily on a concurrent discussion of heart disease.

dition of all the other degenerative diseases. It is particularly dangerous in that under high pressures, an artery in the brain may burst, causing a type of stroke called a cerebrovascular hemorrhage.

ATHEROSCLEROSIS

To live and do its job, each of the body's millions of cells needs to have nutrients brought to it via the blood supply. The heart does the pumping to get the blood there, and the arteries carry the blood from the heart to the cells in every part of the body. To keep all the body cells alive and healthy, the arteries have to remain open and unclogged. If some of the arteries become clogged for any reason, the body cells that are served by these arteries will soon die for lack of oxygen and other nutrients. Atherosclerosis is a disease that clogs the body's arteries, just like rust clogs water pipes in the house.

In atherosclerosis diseased patches, called plaques, develop within the arteries. Over a period of years these plaques may grow so large as to block off an artery entirely. Often before a plaque gets large enough to block the artery in which it is growing, it will break open and spill fragments of festering material into the bloodstream. These fragments may be carried away by the blood only to block another smaller artery someplace downstream. A fragment may block the artery all by itself, if it is large and bulky enough, or it may just act as a core around which a blood clot may grow until the blood clot becomes big enough to block the artery. In any case the result is the same. An artery becomes blocked and the cells which are served by the artery are threatened with death.

Your heart is a muscle that pumps blood throughout your body by regular muscular contractions. Like other body muscles, your heart muscle needs its own supply of blood to stay alive and remain pumping. Arteries called coronary arteries branch off from the main artery coming from the heart and carry a supply of blood around the outside of the heart and down into the heart muscle itself. Coronary arteries, just like any other kind of arteries, can develop atherosclerosis and become clogged. If one of the main coronary arteries becomes blocked by a growing or broken plaque, the muscle cells in the part of the heart supplied by that artery may die of oxygen and nutrient starvation. If this happens to you, you will have experienced a heart attack.

But atherosclerosis can cause blockages in any artery, not just the coronary arteries; therefore, it can also cause the death of cells in other parts of the body. If you develop a block in some of the arteries leading into your brain, it is very likely that some of your brain cells will die. If this happens, you will experience a type of stroke called a cerebral infarction. If you develop a block in arteries leading into your arms or legs, then cell death in your arms or legs is likely to occur. This often leads to gangrene and can even cause the loss of an arm or a leg. The long and short of atherosclerosis is this: It is an extremely dangerous disease and can cause you to lose parts of your body or even your life.

Atherosclerosis is fundamental to both heart disease and stroke. Generally speaking, it is impossible for you to have a heart attack or stroke unless you have first had atherosclerosis for a long time. When a person dies of a heart attack, we seldom think to ourselves: That person died of atherosclerosis. But in a very real sense death was caused by atherosclerosis, because without arterial plaque growth, it is unlikely that the heart attack would have occurred.

The amount of money poured into the treatment of heart disease in this country is truly incredible. Literally billions of dollars are spent by ordinary Americans every year to pay for the cost of their heart attacks. Ironically, no matter how much money one spends repairing a damaged heart, the atherosclerosis that caused all the trouble is still there. Heart troubles will not go away until the atherosclerosis that is the root of the troubles goes away. A first heart attack will likely be followed by another heart attack or by a stroke, by high blood pressure, or by any number of complications.

Fortunately, anyone who cares about himself or his family does not have to see himself or his loved ones die of a heart attack or wind up in a hospital in the intensive care section. There is now convincing evidence that atherosclerosis can be prevented and that the heart attack or stroke that it would cause can be prevented as well. And what is more important for most of us (since most of us already have some degree of atherosclerosis), it may be reversed.

Early Work Was in Heart Disease

Our early understanding of atherosclerosis grew out of our study of heart disease. Heart disease has been a major health problem in this country since the beginning of the century. But it was only after World War II that the health machinery in this country was powerful enough to try to do something about it. In those days the importance of atherosclerosis was not completely realized. It was not generally understood, for example, that atherosclerosis caused not only heart disease but also stroke and perhaps other of the degenerative diseases as well. So, although heart disease was carefully studied, atherosclerosis and the other degenerative diseases were not so carefully studied; their investigation all took a back seat to heart disease. The fact that the degenerative diseases were all closely related was not generally known, and as a result, these diseases were studied as distinct, separate diseases.

The first heart studies after World War II were the beginning of our modern understanding of heart disease. They not only told us a lot about heart disease but also slowly led us into a better understanding of atherosclerosis.

One of the first important studies was begun at the University of Minnesota in 1947 by Dr. Ancel Keys. In 1947 the causes of heart disease were not known. Many people believed that heart disease was more prevalent among the wealthy than among the poor, but this was far from an established fact. There were few established facts, and what Dr. Keys needed was some facts. So in the winter of 1947 Dr. Keys and his associates carefully picked 281 Minnesota businessmen in their 40s and 50s who would become part of what was destined to be a fifteen year study of heart disease.

Dr. Keys knew that as the years went by some of these men would have heart attacks, some would not. He wanted to find out what was different about the men who had heart attacks as compared to those who avoided them. Each year for the next fifteen years those men would come to the University of Minnesota for a complete medical examination. The medical information for those men who suffered heart attacks over the years could thus be compared with the medical records of those men who did not to find the differences for which he was looking.

Early in the study Dr. Keys found two big differences. The biggest difference was in the amount of cholesterol in the blood. It was found that a man who has a very high level of a substance called cholesterol in his blood is much more likely to have a heart attack than a man who has a low level. The fact that cholesterol might somehow be involved with causing heart attacks was a surprise. Cholesterol is a very important body chemical that is used in many ways, including making bile for digestion and even in making the sex hormones. It was surprising that such an important chemical, which the body itself produces, should cause any problems. The other difference that Dr. Keys found was in blood pressure: A man who has high blood pressure is also much more likely to have a heart attack than one who does not.

Now, of course, just because Dr. Keys noticed a difference in blood pressure and cholesterol did not mean that he could jump to the conclusion that high blood pressure and high cholesterol levels cause heart disease. After all, it was certainly possible that some other factors were the cause of heart disease, and that high blood pressure and high cholesterol are just two of possibly many bodily disturbances caused by such other unisolated factors. Today we believe we know what the answer is. We believe today that cholesterol is indeed a causing factor by itself, whereas high blood pressure is simply one of the bodily disturbances resulting primarily from the same underlying factors that produce heart disease. (More about high blood pressure later.) But neither Dr. Keys nor anyone else was sure about this at that time. His study was just the first of many studies begun in that time period.

Other researchers throughout the world set out on similar experiments shortly after Ancel Keys started his Minnesota study. A 12-year study was started in 1948 by the Public Health Service in Framingham, Massachusetts,[8] using a total of 5,209 multiage adults of both sexes. Again the cholesterol level in the blood was found to be the most important factor for predicting that a person might develop heart disease. Ancel Keys himself later engineered a massive study involving more than 12,000 people from seven different countries [9] to see if the worldwide results were any different from his Minnesota results. Here, Dr. Keys found that fats in the blood also correlated with a high incidence of heart disease.

Everybody has fats of different kinds in his blood, just as everybody has cholesterol in his blood. But Dr. Keys' seven-country study showed that when the levels of fat and cholesterol are both high, the chances of a heart attack are suddenly much greater. Other studies have reached the same conclusion. A four-year study involving 3,182 men in San Francisco [10] showed that men whose cholesterol and fat levels were both high had five times as great a chance of suffering a heart attack as men who had low levels for both cholesterol and fat.

The Low Fat/Low Cholesterol Idea

The results of many experiments in the 1950s and 1960s showed for certain that men with high fat and high cholesterol in their blood were bad heart risks. It was soon discovered that there was a link between how much cholesterol and fat one ate in his food and the levels of cholesterol and fat one had in his blood.

Cholesterol is a chemical that you can find only in animal products like cheese, eggs, milk, meat, and fish. All animal products contain cholesterol, some things more than others, but no plant products such as vegetables and fruit contain cholesterol. We in the United States are big meat eaters; we are big egg eaters; we are big cheese eaters, and big milk drinkers. All these foods contain cholesterol. On top of that, our diet is also very high in fats. Fats are not only the fat on the meat that we eat, they are also the cooking oils, the butter, the cream, and the shortening that we eat. Most vegetables have only a little bit of fat, but nuts, avocados, and olives are vegetable products that have a lot of fat. These are all things we Americans love. Believe it or not, the average American gets almost half (42 percent) of his food calories from fats alone. Other countries with high heart disease rates are just about the same. Almost half their food calories come from fats, and their cholesterol intake is high.

Thus, not only are men who have high blood levels of fat

and cholesterol prone to heart disease but so also are men who have high food levels of fat and cholesterol prone to heart disease. For many researchers, that could mean only one thing: Heart disease is caused by a *diet* high in fat and cholesterol. If indeed high fat/high cholesterol food causes heart disease, then the way to prevent heart disease is simply to adopt a low cholesterol/low fat diet.

But there are good scientific reasons for wanting more proof that low cholesterol/low fat foods will prevent heart disease. There were many people who thus would not completely embrace the low fat/low cholesterol idea until a full-scale experiment could be run showing beyond a doubt that if put on low fat/low cholesterol diets then indeed their chances of heart disease would lessen.

This is such an easy experiment to perform and so conclusive that one would expect many experimenters to have jumped at the chance to conduct it. But a quirk of fate having to do with unsaturated fats (which is discussed later) *versus* saturated fats beclouded and confused everything for years, and the needed experiments were slow in coming. But come they eventually did; in the meantime, a great deal of other indirect evidence was being compiled which was capable in itself of establishing the validity of the low cholesterol/low fat diet concept.

Primitive Populations: Indirect Evidence

It is an accident of civilization that the more advanced a culture is, the more fat and cholesterol its people tend to eat. Advanced countries have more animal meat to eat, and the animal meat in advanced countries contains far more fat than wild animal meat. Primitive * people on the other hand are more likely to be near-vegetarians. They generally

---

* We are using the word primitive to describe groups of people who do not have the technology required to perform any significant food processing or mass production of specific food products.

have to be, because without modern technology, it is difficult to have meat much of the time.

If it is true that high fat and high cholesterol diets cause heart disease, then we should expect to see very little heart disease in all those primitive countries that have low fat/low cholesterol diets. And that is exactly what we do find.

In 25 cultures examined [102] in which the people had low fat and low cholesterol diets, no example of a high incidence of heart disease was found. It should be pointed out that primitive people often have very little fat and cholesterol in their diets compared to us. While our diet is 42 percent fat, theirs is often less than 10 percent fat. That is quite a difference. A diet with that little fat is practically unheard of in this country, and it is quite difficult to obtain such a meal in any restaurant. Let us consider a couple of the primitive peoples that have been studied.*

Practically all of the lower half of Africa is populated by a race of people known as the Bantu. The Bantus give us an ideal group of people to study because their diet is a primitive low fat/low cholesterol one, and there are so many Bantus to study: more than 50 million of them. As you might expect from what has already been stated, heart disease is almost nonexistent among Bantus. The Nkana Nune Hospital is a large modern hospital serving Bantus in southern Africa. During a 5-year period in the 1950s, not a single Bantu died of heart disease in this hospital. The hospital also operates a small wing for Europeans in the area. Only a tenth of the patients in this hospital are Europeans, and yet during the same 5-year period 23 Europeans died of heart disease in that institution.[11]

---

* Eskimos have often been quoted as an example of a *high* fat culture with relatively little heart disease. However, according to a recent study (reference 103), Eskimos derive approximately 23 percent of their calories from fat. This is only about half the fat that is consumed by the average American.

The Bantus are not yet in the mainstream of Western civilization, so that their ways of living and eating are still the same as they have been for thousands of years. Their diet is only about 10 percent fat, and they eat very little cholesterol a day—about a fifth of what an average American eats. The amount of fat and cholesterol in the blood of people who were tested, and who were in excellent health, was so low [12] that it would be considered abnormal by most American doctors.

The situation with a group of New Guinea natives studied by Whyte [13] is essentially the same. These aborigines eat only a fifth as much cholesterol and less than a quarter as much fat as the average American. As a result fat and cholesterol levels in their blood are low throughout their lives, and heart disease is quite rare among these people. In a study done in the late 1950s, autopsies were performed on 600 New Guineans who had died for various reasons, to determine in every case the exact cause of death. Out of these 600 cases, only one death could be attributed to heart disease. Another interesting finding was that the New Guinean's blood pressure does not increase as he grows older. In fact, around middle age his diastolic blood pressure drops 10 points. In the United States, blood pressure goes up as we age, worsening our problems with heart disease and strokes.

In Ecuador the results are the same.[14] In primitive groups around the world—whether in Africa, New Guinea, or Ecuador—the results are always the same: Low fat/low cholesterol means low incidence of heart disease. There is no counter-example to this—no example of people with a low fat/low cholesterol diet who reveal any significant incidence of heart disease.

Although not a primitive people, such as those mentioned above, the Japanese elect a very low fat/low cholesterol diet throughout most of their homeland. In fact, even with the strong American influence since the war, most Japanese still subsist on a diet containing only 10 percent fat and consume far less cholesterol than the average European or American. Consequently, the heart disease rate in Japan is only a ninth of what it is here in the United States.[9]

It is still possible of course that it is merely coincidence that the low fat/low cholesterol populations we have studied are free of heart disease. They might be free of heart disease only because they have strong genes that protect them. That is, it is possible that all those people studied are *naturally immune* to heart disease, and that it is this natural immunity rather than their food that saves them from heart disease.

It is possible to check out this idea. If indeed natural immunity rather than consumed food is responsible for protecting these people from heart disease, then one would expect them to be free of heart disease no matter what their diets happen to be.

Ancel Keys, in the late 1950s, studied Japanese populations in three different environments.[15] He studied a group of Japanese who had remained in Japan, a second group who had migrated to Hawaii, and a third group who had migrated to Los Angeles. As mentioned, the diet in Japan is a low cholesterol and fat one. The Hawaiians' diet, on the other hand, tends to be an intermediate cholesterol and fat diet,* while the Los Angeles diet is typically American: high cholesterol and fat diet. It was found that the Japanese group in Japan had a very low incidence of heart disease. The Japanese group in Hawaii, on the other hand,

---

* In most diets if fat is high, so is cholesterol. If fat is low, so is cholesterol. It is unusual to find people employing a diet which is high in one and low in the other. The reason for this is that high-fat diets typically come from eating lots of meat; lots of meat invariably also brings lots of cholesterol, since cholesterol is only available in animal products. On the other hand, to cut down on fat, people usually must cut down on meat, which in turn cuts down on cholesterol.

had a significantly higher incidence of heart disease, while the Japanese group in Los Angeles evidenced a rate of heart disease equal to that suffered by Americans. This study showed that protection from heart disease, at least among the Japanese, does not stem from natural immunity. There was obviously something happening to the "displaced" Japanese to erase his protection, and once again protection seemed to be related to diet.

Animal Experiments: Additional Evidence

Studies conducted with populations such as the Japanese, as well as the primitive groups, added very important pieces of evidence to support the idea that dietary fat and cholesterol are causes of heart disease. But none of these studies were direct enough. Not one of them directly showed how you could take a perfectly healthy heart and give it heart disease by diet alone. Although it is nearly impossible to do laboratory experiments on people, for moral and practical reasons, it is easy to do laboratory experiments on animals. Even though an animal does not have exactly the same body chemistry as a human, it is still very important to see whether or not heart disease can be caused in animals solely by introducing a high fat/high cholesterol diet.

During the 20 years between 1950 and 1970, therefore, many laboratory experiments were conducted to find out if diet can cause heart disease in animals. In experimenting with animals to find possible correlations to human beings, it is usually important to pick animals that are as much like man as possible. A snail, for example, has a metabolism which is so different from a man's that it would be very hard to draw any conclusions about man from studying snails, except perhaps in the area of the most basic of biochemical processes. On the other hand, a rat is a lot more like a man than a snail. That is, it has bones, skin, legs, and internal organs like a man. Thus the rat is often studied in the place of man when it is impossible to study the human being. However, the laboratory animal most often used when it is important that the lab animal be like a man as much as possible is the monkey.

A fatal heart attack was produced in a rhesus monkey for the first time in 1959. The heart failure was produced strictly by feeding the monkey a high fat/high cholesterol diet. The diet was very much like what many Americans consume every day. It was about 42 percent fat and about a 50th of an ounce of cholesterol per day.[16] After two years on the diet the monkey had developed the characteristic yellow outcroppings (called *xanthomas*) on his skin, which showed that its atherosclerosis was already well developed. After two and a half years the fatal heart attack happened. The attack was massive, involving about half of his left heart muscle. The heart and the coronary arteries looked just like a human heart looks after such an attack. The heart showed many areas of cell death, and the arteries were filled with plaques. It should be pointed out that rhesus monkeys do not have heart attacks under normal circumstances. On ordinary monkey chow, a rhesus monkey will never have a heart attack.

Since that time the experiment has been repeated many times by many researchers on different animals. The results are always the same: High fat and high cholesterol produce heart disease. In animal experiments, therefore, the evidence is as direct as you can possibly expect. If you take an animal with a clean, healthy heart and feed him a high fat/high cholesterol diet, his heart will become diseased and fail.

Atherosclerosis: A Growing Understanding

During the 1950s and 1960s the public began to appreciate the importance of atherosclerosis as a cause of heart disease. It soon became apparent that fat and cholesterol were doing

How to Solve the Problem   31

bodily harm by causing clogged arteries: Or in other words, by causing atherosclerosis.

Although there are many details that are still cloudy, the main picture of how fat and cholesterol cause atherosclerosis is now known. The next few paragraphs are devoted to briefly relating how atherosclerosis comes about. This explanation is very important because it builds the background necessary to understand other degenerative diseases as well.

Figure 2 below is a cutaway of a large human artery. This picture shows that the artery has several layers like the layers in a high quality garden hose, and it shows the names of these various layers. The figure displays the layers as smooth sheaths of material. However, in reality things are much different. Every part of the artery is actually a network of cells, much like a honeycomb is a network of cells that hold honey. For example, if we were to look very

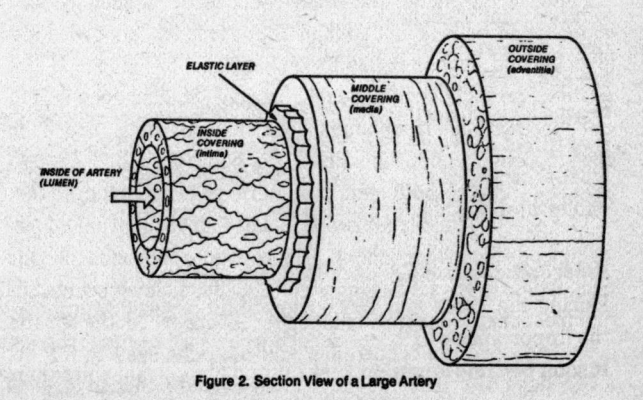

Figure 2. Section View of a Large Artery

carefully at the inside layer (*intima*) of the artery, we would see that it consists of many separate cells fitted together like a jigsaw puzzle. Figure 3 shows how the cells of the intima fit together to form the inside layer.

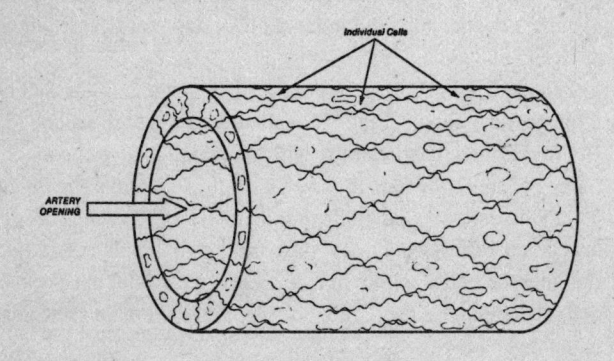

Figure 3. The Intima of an Artery

Like the intima, all the other parts of the artery are also made up of cells. Each part of the artery has its own kind of cells, and each cell has its own special job to do. If the cell has the right working environment, then it does its job well; in turn, the body stays healthy and strong. But if its working environment is ruined, the cell will fail. If enough cells fail then the body gets sick, perhaps sick enough to die.

The story of atherosclerosis relates the ruination of arterial cellular environment and the consequences of this ruin. Atherosclerosis begins when the elastic layer surrounding the intima becomes damaged. Damage to the elastic layer is a common occurrence and happens even in infants a few days old. It is not yet known why the elastic layer is so easily broken or fragmented. Perhaps it breaks because the artery is twisted, flexed, or compacted. But whatever the reason, it happens all the time. These breaks heal and leave insignificant scars that do no damage so long as the blood's cholesterol and fats are at low levels. However, if these levels are high, then cholesterol and fat can irritate the ruptured elastic layer, and begin a sequence of fateful events.

When the intima cells in the ruptured area come in contact with cholesterol and fat particles in their vicinity, they automatically begin to swallow up these particles to get rid of them. As more and more particles are fed in by the blood to replace the ones taken in by these cells, the cells begin to multiply to be able to handle these new fat and cholesterol particles. Soon they have multiplied and spread so much that they completely surround the elastic layer's broken area. By this time the cells in the vicinity of the break may have taken in so much fat and cholesterol particles that they may be swollen to several times their original size. Their appearance at this time takes on a foamy look, and, appropriately, they are called "foam" cells.

At this stage the injury is called a "fatty streak" and can be seen on the artery's inside wall. This streak could remain indefinitely in the artery, causing no harm. The foam cells are still living cells; they have all the chemicals in them necessary to dispose of the fat and cholesterol particles they contain and in time return to their normal size. If the fat and cholesterol in the blood are brought down to low levels, this will in fact happen, and no harm will have been done.

If, however, the levels remain high, then the foam cells will continue to take in particles until at last the cells begin to burst, spilling their contents into the surrounding area. The burst cells cause the body to begin a protective process called *fibrosis*, whereby connective tissue—the sort of tissue that makes up ligaments—begins to grow through and around the damaged area to seal it off from the rest of the artery. Soon the process of fibrosis will convert the fatty streak into a full-grown plaque, called a *fibrolipid* plaque, which by then may extend like an abcessed sore clear up into the adventitia covering of the artery. Figure 4 is a diagram of what the cross section of a healthy artery should

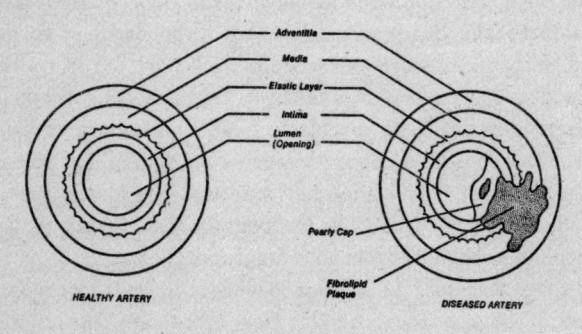

Figure 4. Cross Section of Healthy Artery and Cross Section of Artery with Fibrolipid Plaque

look like, as compared to one in which a fibrolipid plaque has developed.

This plaque will eventually be sealed off from the blood flowing through the artery by a cap of fibrous material, and with the cap in place, the plaque is called a *pearly* plaque. No more blood will reach the plaque's interior from the blood flowing through the artery, but blood can reach the interior of the plaque through tiny new arteries that the body sends down from the adventitia into the plaque. With the presence of more blood and more fat and cholesterol from the inside this time, new foam cells will form and die, spilling their contents into the plaque. By this time the plaque is full of dead material, the normal bodily processes of sealing off the affected area do not function properly, and the plaque becomes gradually free to degenerate, until it, too, arrives at the point of bursting.

When the bursting of the plaque finally occurs, blood from the artery rushes in and a blood clot forms around the ruptured area. Debris from the rupture may now circulate through the bloodstream, forming the core of numerous other blood clots. If the debris stays attached to the ruptured area, the clot that forms may be so large as to completely close off the artery, or at least greatly reduce the artery's opening. If the clot does not kill the person at this stage, the body will work hard to grow new arteries or new "canals" through the artery's blocked-off part. Plaques may thus become "canalized" with new vessels, which to some extent compensate for the reduced blood flow caused by the plaque. Unfortunately, the new vessels tend to have poorly developed media and adventitia and tend to rupture easily. At this last stage the person so afflicted is not only loaded with plaques but also loaded with fragile new vessels which are unpredictable and easily ruptured. Ruptures of new vessels such as these appear to be responsible for many fatal heart attacks.

Reversal of Atherosclerosis: A Big Second Chance

A large majority of the readers of this book already have atherosclerosis. Some may not have had any symptoms yet and probably are unaware that they have it. Some, however, have already survived their first or second heart attack and are very aware of their atherosclerosis. But no matter how bad the atherosclerosis is, there is mounting evidence that much can be done to reverse it and clean up the clogged arteries.

Naturally one is better off keeping one's arteries clean in the first place rather than cleaning up dirty arteries later. But in either case, whether one is keeping clean arteries clean or cleaning up dirty ones, the thing to be done is the same: namely cholesterol and fats must be reduced in one's food intake.

The research going on in the area of reversing atherosclerosis is still in its early stages. But the results of research done so far are highly promising and encouraging. The most conclusive work to date was done in 1970 and 1971 with rhesus monkeys. The object of the rhesus experiments was to induce atherosclerosis in an experimental colony of animals by introducing a high fat/high cholesterol diet and then reverse the diet for a period of time to see how much the atherosclerosis regressed during that time.

M. L. Armstrong and his associates fed 30 rhesus monkeys a high fat/high cholesterol diet for nearly a year and a half.[27] After this length of time, 10 of the animals were picked to be "baseline" animals to see how much atherosclerosis this diet was generating. The coronary arteries of these 10 baseline animals were examined, and as expected, they were extensively atherosclerotic. On the average, the coronary arteries were more than 50 percent closed by atherosclerotic plaques. The remaining 20 animals were then fed a low cholesterol diet for 40 months to see if these plaques could be reversed. Ten of these animals were fed very little fat (4 percent) in addition to zero cholesterol, whereas for the other 10 this same zero cholesterol diet was heavily supplemented with unsaturated fat (40 percent). Armstrong was thus trying to find out not only what effect is created by a reversal to a diet low in both fat and cholesterol, but also what effect is created by a diet that is low in cholesterol but high in fats of the unsaturated variety.

At the end of the 40 months the arteries of all 20 low-cholesterol animals were examined. It was found that the 10 animals on the diet low in both fat and cholesterol had reduced their plaques to about a fourth the amount shown by the 10 baseline animals which had not had any reversal diet at all. The 10 animals assigned diets with no cholesterol but high in unsaturated fats also had their plaques greatly reversed; however, there still remained 50 percent more plaques than produced by the low-fat diet.

This experiment showed for the first time that atherosclerosis can be reversed by the same low cholesterol/low fat diet that must be used to prevent it. The experiment also showed that a diet low in cholesterol but high in fats—even unsaturated fats—is not nearly as good at reversing atherosclerosis as a diet low in both fats and cholesterol.

Other experiments on rhesus monkeys done by Tucker and his associates showed similar results: Atherosclerosis can be reversed by switching to low fat/low cholesterol foods.[28] The same kind of experiments have not been conducted with human beings; however, with all that is known today, and in the opinion of this book's authors, it is beyond doubt that human atherosclerosis is reversed just as dramatically as the atherosclerosis in the rhesus monkeys by a switch to low fat/low cholesterol foods.

A Backward Look at Some of Our Mistakes in Atherosclerosis

The notion of the low fat/low cholesterol diet for the prevention and treatment of atherosclerosis is a simple one. Yet this concept was not arrived at overnight; along the way a number of misconceptions were encountered, and mistakes were made in the treatment and prevention of atherosclerosis and heart disease. Since some of these mistakes are still being practiced, it is wise to know something about them.

Unsaturated Fats: The Great Misunderstanding

As previously discussed, the relation was found very early in the game (about 1950) between the amount of cholesterol one has in his blood and heart disease: the more blood cholesterol, the more heart disease. At about the same time, a great misunderstanding happened in the search for the answers to the heart disease question. It was found that if a person ate large amounts of the unsaturated fats (such as corn and safflower oil), the amount of cholesterol in his blood would go down. Even though the connection between cholesterol and heart disease was still questionable at that time, it seemed reasonable to get people to start substituting unsaturated fats for the saturated ones (such as animal fat and butter fat) that people ordinarily were eating. In the 1950s a great interest in unsaturated fats was thus ignited that has carried down to this day. Unsaturated fats seemed like the miracle answer to heart disease. Instead of giving up cholesterol-bearing products such as eggs, shell fish, and lots of steak, all we would have to do is replace a portion of our saturated fats with unsaturated ones. Soon everyone got on the bandwagon from the margarine manufacturers to the American Heart Association: Eat more unsaturated fats and get less heart disease.

It is sad but true that unsaturated fats were not the simple answer for which everyone had hoped. The facts were long in being sorted out, and in the meantime, the main thrust of research on heart disease went off in the wrong direction. Many studies were done on different kinds of diets in the years that followed, and nearly all of them included large amounts of unsaturated fats as a basic part of the diet. As a result, tests of truly low-fat diets (all fats, not just saturated ones) on large populations were not emphasized. Money and manpower were thus expended down fruitless lines of research that produced confusing data, and many researchers finally concluded, erroneously, that heart disease has nothing to do with diet, so must be inherited and/or emotional. Even to this day there are important research efforts marching off down the dead-end road of unsaturated fats.

How to Solve the Problem 39

Evidence that unsaturated fats would prevent heart disease was only circumstantial, so to speak, and in the last analysis, this circumstantial evidence has not held up in court. There was certainly plenty of hard evidence on the prevention of heart disease, but it had relatively little to do with unsaturated fats. The major hard facts of the case were these:

1. Wherever and however animals were fed high cholesterol/high fat diets, atherosclerosis and heart disease were sure to follow.
2. All populations studied with diets low in fats and cholesterol were found to be comparatively free of atherosclerosis and heart disease.
3. All populations studied with high heart disease and atherosclerosis rates were found to have:
   a) High amounts of fat and cholesterol in the diets,
   b) High levels of fat and cholesterol in the blood.

Fact 3b implies that a man who has heart disease or who is in the process of developing heart disease is very likely to have high levels of cholesterol in his blood. Suppose then that we were able to invent a drug which would lessen his cholesterol level. Would his heart disease go away or not be produced in the first place? The answer is, we don't know. Although it is tempting to guess that this might be the case, the fact is that from available evidence we simply cannot tell. Such a drug might certainly make some of the cholesterol go out of the blood, but it might also produce widespread side effects, such as perhaps removing this cholesterol from the blood and putting it into the arterial plaques instead! From our previous discussion of cholesterol, plaques, and atherosclerosis, it is clear that this is the last thing we would want to have happen. Such a drug might thus actually accelerate this case of heart disease rather than prevent it or cure it. Indeed, given the fantastic complexity of the arterial metabolic processes (about which we know very little), it would be surprising if our hypothetical drug did not do more damage than good.

The situation with unsaturated fats was exactly the same as the situation with our hypothetical drug. Although eating unsaturated fats made the cholesterol level in the blood go down significantly, there was no evidence that heart disease and atherosclerosis would be prevented or reduced as well. In fact, as time passed, evidence began to accumulate which seemed to show that unsaturated fats might be doing just what was feared the most: transferring cholesterol from the blood into the arterial plaques and other body tissue.

In the rat,[21] in the rabbit,[69] in the rhesus monkey,[22] and in the cebus monkey,[70] the results all pointed in the same direction: A diet high in unsaturated fats did indeed lower blood cholesterol levels, but at the same time it increased the amounts of cholesterol in the arterial plaques, artery wall, liver, and other body tissues. Furthermore, there was no reason to believe that the metabolism of human beings would behave any differently. And there is every reason to believe that such behavior by the cholesterol in the human being could be very dangerous.

Other disturbing things also came to light. Meyer Friedman and his associates in San Francisco showed[71] that unsaturated fats in the diet produced just as much fat blockage in the capillaries as ordinary animal fat, often staying in the bloodstream far longer than ordinary animal fat. In addition, Marvin Bierenbaum and his associates in New Jersey[72] performed an experiment with 200 men who had already had heart attacks; its results indicated that unsaturated fats are no better at protecting such men from further heart attack and death than saturated fats.

Not only was there no evidence that the lowering of cholesterol levels with unsaturated fats was beneficial, there was even evidence to the contrary. Yet the notion of unsaturated fats seemed to hold everyone in a spell, and the reality of the evidence could not pierce through the fog of misundersanding that was created by that single misconstrued discovery that unsaturated fats reduce blood cholesterol. The extent to which the notion of unsaturated fats dominated early thinking can be seen by looking at Table I. This table shows 12 of the most important dietary studies conducted in the 1950s and 1960s. In each of these studies the aim was to see whether or not a cholesterol-lowering diet could in fact reduce heart disease in people. But out of these 12 studies, all but 3 used high fat diets (28 percent to 46 percent of the total calories of the diet were fat) in which unsaturated fats were added to the diet or were substituted for the diet's ordinary animal fats. Of the 3 exceptions (studies 7, 9, and 11), only Morrison's study (study 9) was undeniably based on a low fat/low cholesterol diet. The other two suffered from experimental difficulties that make it difficult to determine exactly how much fat was actually used in the diets. Out of the 12 studies only one can thus be regarded as a truly low fat/low cholesterol study. Except for two dubious studies, all the rest were essentially high fat studies using unsaturated fats in place of or in addition to the animal fats of the normal modern diet. It is a fact that, taken as a body, these 12 studies revealed nothing significant as far as reducing heart disease. In reviewing these 12 studies, Jerome Cornfield at the University of Pittsburgh had this to say: "It seems clear that despite a very considerable scientific effort in these studies and some tantalizing suggestive results, we have no clear-cut, generally accepted answer to the question of whether cholesterol-lowering measures can affect heart disease."

In short, there is no evidence whatever that adding unsaturated fats to our diet will help reduce heart disease, and everywhere we look we run into this fact. But the situation

Table I. TWELVE IMPORTANT DIETARY STUDIES OF THE 1950s AND 1960s

Study	Number of Patients — Dieters	Number of Patients — Normals	Length of Study	Dieter's Percentage Drop in Blood Cholesterol	Percent in Fats of Diet
1. Leren [18] (1970)	206	206	5 yrs.	18	39
2. Turpeinen [74] (1968)	313	241	6 yrs.	13	31
3. Dayton [20] et al. (1969)	424	422	5–8 yrs.	19	39
4. Bierenbaum [72] et al. (1967)	100	100	7 yrs.	9	28
5. Rinzler [73] (1968)	941	457	Up to 10 yrs.	13	33
6. Hood [76] et al. (1965)	112	112	5–17 yrs.	16	45
7. Nelson [77] (1956)	170	0	3–6 yrs.	15	No data
8. Hanson [78] et al. (1962)	133	132	Up to 17 mo.	13	36
9. Morrison [75] et al. (1960)	50	50	12 yrs.	29	15
10. Rose [79] et al. (1965)	28	26	2 yrs.	8	35
11. Ball [80] (1965)	123	129	Average 3 yrs.	17	No data
12. Morris [19] (1968)	199	194	2–7 yrs.	16	46

with the low fat/low cholesterol diet is entirely different. The original hard evidence listed on page 39 points directly at the low fat/low cholesterol diet as the means for preventing heart disease, and no evidence has ever been uncovered that points even mildly to the contrary. In addition, Morrison's study shows us directly that the low fat/low cholesterol diet will ameliorate heart disease. It is an interesting fact that even though not a drop of unsaturated fat was added to the dieters' food in Morrison's study, nevertheless, Morrison's low fat/low cholesterol diet produced by far the largest decrease in blood cholesterol of any of the other 12 studies in Table I.

And except for the study by Hood,[*] Morrison's study also was the only study that showed any significant difference in the death rates between people who ate the cholesterol-lowering diet, and people who ate normally. In Morrison's case the results were impressive. Morrison used two groups of 50 subjects each, all of whom had already suffered a heart attack, and all of whom therefore had a relatively poor chance to live as long as the normal population. One group, the control group, ate normally. But the other group, the experimental one, was placed on a low fat (15 percent)/low cholesterol diet. After 12 years, every single person in the control group had died, but at that same time, 38 percent of the experimental group had survived.

But despite all this evidence, much of which came to us years ago, the unsaturated fat concept persisted. To this day, many researchers are still using the shaky tenets of unsaturated fats. Even now a large Federal study is being launched [81] in which heart disease control is being attempted using methods which rely, among other things,

[*] Although Hood's results seem to show that people die more frequently on a normal diet than they do on his cholesterol-lowering diet using lots of unsaturated fats, his results appear to be clouded by difficulties in experimental design.

on large amounts of unsaturated fats in the diet (30 to 35 percent total calories from fats alone). From all that we know at this time, it appears likely that this study will ultimately arrive at the conclusion that there is not much difference in the likelihood of early death for a person using the study's heart disease control methods than for a normal person; a pretty inconclusive result, given the amount of money (100 million) being spent. On the other hand, if the fat levels in the study were pushed down to 10 percent or less, the conclusiveness of the situation would probably do an abrupt turnabout. In this case it appears likely that the ultimate conclusion would be that a person using the study's heart disease control methods would be much less likely to experience early death than a normal person.

Emotional Stress: A Cause for Ulcers but Not Heart Disease

A school of thought flourishes that believes that emotional stress—involving anger, aggressiveness, anxiety, and so forth—is responsible for heart attacks. This school of thinking began in the mid-1950s, and the idea that tension and stress were responsible for heart attacks spread quickly throughout the country. According to some followers there are basically two types of personalities: type A personality, prone to heart atttacks, and type B personality, resistant to heart attacks. The type A man could be characterized as aggressive, driving, and domineering, whereas the type B man could be characterized as relaxed, satisfied, and passive. The doctor who believes in this personality type theory has ways of diagnosing whether a person is type A or type B by watching his behavior while answering questions. In the extreme, the type A person might talk rapidly and explosively, clenching his jaw muscles and his hands, for example, while the type B person might be relaxed and answer more slowly.

The idea that stress caused heart attacks was very popular and, even today, still has some legal standing. For instance, in workmen's compensation cases, if a doctor testifies that the stresses of a man's job caused him to have a heart attack, the government must pay him compensation.

But what data exist to tell us whether or not stress has any effect on heart disease? Up to the present time situations that have been studied, which might in some way be thought of as stressful, have failed to cause increases in the incidence of heart disease. For this reason the notion that stress causes heart disease has lost much of its glamor.

Many animal experiments have been performed, for example, in which animals were subjected to all sorts of stressful situations. Roosters were tested in a situation where they were repeatedly and unavoidably subjected to electrical shocks for long periods during their lives.[23] Upon surgical examination the "shocked" roosters revealed no more heart disease than the ones not subjected to shock. Rabbits[24] were subjected to the stresses of extreme cold. When the rabbits were killed and examined there was no more heart disease in the cold rabbits than there was in the warm rabbits.

Stress is supposed to be greater for men in upper executive posts than men in blue-collar jobs. To test the idea that this form of stress might cause heart attacks, a five-year study of 270,000 Bell Telephone employees was run.[25] Dr. Hinkle, who ran the study, said that the results "didn't come out the way I anticipated. Heart disease is not greatly influenced by the tensions of adult life in an industrial society." Results showed that top management men not only did not have more heart disease than blue-collar men, they actually had less.

One might think that living under the Nazi occupation in World War II would cause the sort of stresses that the stress people claim will cause heart disease. But it was found, for example, in a review of 24,546 autopsies performed in

Austria,[26] that there were eight times as many heart attacks in the postwar year of 1948 as there were in the wartime occupation year of 1944. (We might note here that after the war the diet of the Austrians grew to include a great deal of fat and cholesterol, whereas during the war the diet was a very skimpy, low fat/low cholesterol one.)

So far it has been simply impossible to find a stressful situation that will cause heart attacks under laboratory conditions. All the evidence seems to show that stress is, at best, only a minor factor in the cause of heart disease. This notion has thus to some extent been abandoned by researchers and medical practitioners alike, although from time to time we still encounter someone espousing the idea of stress-caused heart disease.

Cholesterol-lowering Drugs: A Dismal Picture

We described above a hypothetical drug for lowering blood-cholesterol levels. We asked ourselves the question: Will this cholesterol-lowering drug reduce heart disease? And we saw that the answer was: We cannot tell from all the data we now have, but in view of the complexity of the body's cell metabolism in the artery, it seems likely that a cholesterol-lowering drug would do more harm than good.

Despite this likelihood, when a number of drugs such as our hypothetical one were actually found that would lower cholesterol levels in the blood, there was a great deal of interest in the medical community to try them out. As a result in recent years cholesterol-lowering drugs were tried by many physicians on their patients and on themselves in the hopes that heart disease could thereby be prevented or cured. Unfortunately the insight gained from such attempts was anything but encouraging. One drug, triparanol, which received a great deal of early attention, not only did not reduce heart disease but it evidently caused cataracts and other toxic effects in its users who included many physicians.

How to Solve the Problem 47

The biggest study of cholesterol-lowering drugs, which is now nearly complete, and from which many preliminary results were obtained, was devised by the National Heart and Lung Institute.[82,83] This carefully designed study, the Coronary Drug Project (CDP), required more than four years simply to select the 8,341 participants in the study. The participants selected were men aged 30 to 64 who had already had a heart attack. Fundamentally, the object of CDP was to determine if the life expectancies of these men would be increased or decreased by any of the following four drugs:

1. Conjugated Estrogens
2. DT 4
3. Nicotinic Acid
4. Clofibrate

In performing this experiment, the total population of men was divided into five groups, one group for each of the four drugs, and a fifth group which was to take no drugs at all, but was to act instead as control group, against which comparisons of the effectiveness of the other groups could be made.

By the end of the third year of the 5-year CDP experiment, the DT 4 group was discontinued altogether. Comparisons showed that the death rate of the people taking DT 4 was nearly 20% higher than the death rate for the control group. This happened *despite the fact that DT 4 did indeed lower cholesterol* (by 12%) and it even lowered blood fats (by more than 15%). At this same time, half of the subjects taking estrogen were also discontinued from the study * because their death rates were also higher than that experienced by the control group, by about 30%. Data on nicotinic

---

* The estrogen group was divided into two parts. A group taking 5 mg. of the drug, and a group taking 2-½ mg. The 5 mg. group was the one dropped from the study.

acid and clofibrate are still incomplete, but early evidence is not encouraging, and it appears that difficulty will be found with these drugs as well.

The results of the CDP experiment have been anything but promising. The view that a cholesterol-lowering drug is likely to do more harm than good has so far been reinforced by the CDP experiment results, and future results are not likely to change this situation very much. The thing that we have learned from cholesterol-lowering drugs is this: They *do* lower cholesterol; they *do not* reduce heart disease.

DIABETES

"Diabetes" is a medical word used to describe several different diseases, but by far the most common form, and the one we will talk about, is "sugar diabetes." Sugar diabetes is an extremely serious illness that sometimes appears in children, but usually waits till the middle-age years or later to appear. The sure sign of sugar diabetes is high levels of sugar in the blood and sugar in the urine. Some of the symptoms of sugar diabetes are: overwhelming thirst and appetite and rapid loss of body weight and body water. In severe cases, if sugar diabetes is left untreated, its victim will rapidly lose weight, grow extremely weak, pass into a diabetic coma, and die.

Even under careful treatment the victim of sugar diabetes (or simply diabetes, as we shall hereafter call it) has always had a dismal future. The diabetic has a much higher than normal susceptibility to heart disease and atherosclerosis. He may become progressively blinded by the disease in addition to suffering from palsy, impotency, boils, and progressively impaired hearing. In short, it has been an extremely dangerous and distasteful disease, even under careful treatment.

How to Solve the Problem   49

Fortunately, like atherosclerosis, diabetes can be prevented and reversed in a great many people. But like atherosclerosis, the road to understanding the prevention of diabetes has been a long and rocky one.

For more than 80 years it was thought by nearly every researcher that diabetes was caused by a failure of the pancreas. The pancreas, a large organ located just behind the stomach, produces several chemicals that are needed by the body to extract energy and nutrients from food. More than 80 years ago Von Mering and Minkowski showed that all of diabetes' symptoms could be created in a dog by destroying its pancreas. They showed that the destruction of other organs did not cause diabetic symptoms, but the destruction of the pancreas always caused these symptoms.

For 30 years after the Von Mering-Minkowski experiments, scientists the world over tried to discover what ingredient the pancreas produced that, when taken away from the body, resulted in diabetes. In 1922 two researchers, F. G. Banting, a Canadian, and J. J. R. Macleod, a Scot, finally succeeded in isolating a pancreatic extract that would prevent the sure symptoms of diabetes from developing, even in a dog with a destroyed pancreas. Banting and Macleod called their extract insulin, and insulin became the century's miracle discovery.

Today we know a lot about insulin. It is a hormone secreted into the blood by the pancreas. It is in some way vital to the burning of sugar in the body. Sugar, a vital source of energy for all cells in the body, is carried to the cells in the blood. Without this sugar in our blood we would die. In fact, if the sugar level in the blood drops even a little bit, we develop a condition called hypoglycemia, which causes fatigue, faintness, nausea, and other symptoms.

Insulin is needed in order for the body's cells to be able to take up and utilize blood sugar. If the insulin is ineffective or absent, sugar will not be taken from the blood by the cells, and the level of sugar will build up to staggering levels. In such a case the kidneys, which are responsible for filtering the blood, become overwhelmed by the high level of sugar, and sugar begins to spill over into the urine.

As soon as insulin was generally available, virtually all diabetes was treated with daily insulin injections. Insulin was very effective at controlling the level of the blood sugar, and almost overnight deaths from diabetic coma in the United States dropped to a very low level. It appeared that the cause of diabetes was clearly known: a defective pancreas. Somehow, people believed, the diabetic's pancreas had stopped producing insulin which, in turn, caused diabetes. To cure diabetes all you had to do, it was believed, was to provide the needed insulin in an artificial way.

Unfortunately, there were a number of disturbing facts emerging about diabetics. Even though diabetics on insulin no longer needed to fear immediate death from diabetic coma, there was a huge class of fearful health complications that plagued them, ranging from blindness to gangrene, as well as severe heart disease. Somehow diabetics, even on insulin which theoretically was all they needed, were far from being healthy.

As years passed the biochemistry of insulin and sugar metabolism became better and better understood. The chemical structure of insulin was completely worked out, and insulin was finally created artificially in the laboratory a few years ago. As the biochemical pathways in the body painstakingly began to be worked out, it became clearer and clearer how immensely complex the whole business of sugar metabolism and other chemical processes are. Literally hundreds of chemicals are involved in the processes, and hormones such as insulin are delicately—and in most cases mysteriously—involved in all of them. Above all it became clear that the simple act of injecting more insulin into the diabetic's bloodstream would create far-reaching implications that were literally impossible to fathom with the state of current knowledge.

Experience was showing us that diabetics were far from getting well, while science was showing us that there was no valid reason why they should be getting well by simply receiving insulin injections.

In 1960 a technological breakthrough occurred. R. S. Yalow and S. A. Berson devised, for the first time, a technique for accurately measuring the amount of insulin present in the blood at any given time.[104] Because of the way in which insulin is transported in the bloodstream, this had not been possible before this time. By the late 1960s, using the Yalow-Berson technique, several remarkable discoveries were made. It was discovered by G. M. Reaven and his associates at Stanford that diabetics often had more insulin present in their blood than nondiabetics.[29,30,31] It was furthermore discovered that a diabetic's pancreas could produce just as much insulin and just as quickly as that of a normal person.

In one stroke, the cherished theory that diabetes is always caused by a defective pancreas was thus swept away. For how could a pancreas be "defective" if it could produce just as much insulin and just as quickly as a normal pancreas, as is very often the case?

Other researchers about the same time [32,131] discovered that the sensitivity of insulin appeared to be significantly decreased in the presence of fats in the blood. Furthermore, it was known that diabetics typically had high levels of fat in their blood.[57,58] Thus many things became clear all at once: Suppose that diabetes were usually caused, not by an absence of insulin, but rather by decreased insulin efficiency in the presence of fat. What would we expect to find then? We would expect to find excessive blood sugar even though for many diabetics there was plenty of insulin around to metabolize it. This we do find.[29,30,31] We would expect to find that injected insulin would be able to metabolize the blood sugar, but not necessarily normalize the diabetic. This we do find.[64,65,66] We would expect that diabetes would correlate strongly with a high level of fats in the blood. This we do find.[57,58,131,132] We would expect that lowering blood fats by any means—diet or drugs—would increase insulin sensitivity and would decrease the severity of the diabetes. This we do find.[32,59,131,133,134]

By the beginning of the 1970s, therefore, it was clear that diabetes was not due to a defective pancreas as had traditionally been thought, but indeed was often connected to the fat levels in the blood and a resulting decreased efficiency of the body's insulin. The natural question then was: Could diabetes be prevented and treated by a low-fat diet, just as heart disease can be prevented and treated by the low fat/low cholesterol diet?

Several studies on the low-fat control of diabetes had already been done in past years, and their results had at once shown the power of the low-fat diet in the control of diabetes. These studies were largely unheeded by the medical profession because they called for dietary procedures that were not compatible with then existing theories about diabetes. Today under the illumination of more facts and a better theoretical picture of diabetes, their importance is obvious.

I. M. Rabinowitch performed the earliest and the largest study of the treatment of diabetes with low fat foods. In 1935 Dr. Rabinowitch reported his findings on 100 insulin-dependent diabetic patients in his clinic in Montreal. His study was a 5-year controlled experiment in which 50 patients were placed on the conventional diabetic diet, and 50 were placed on a new low-fat diet.

The thrust of his results are that the patients on the low-fat diet remarkably reduced their dependence on insulin, while the other patients did not. On the low fat diet 24%

of the patients had ceased using insulin altogether and were normal as shown by lab tests and clinical observation. In addition, the remainder of them had reduced their insulin dependence from an average of 24.6 units of insulin per day to an average of 10.6 units per day.

The other 50 patients, those on the standard diabetic diet, did not fare nearly so well. There was no change in the average insulin dosage for the group over the entire 5-year time span. At the start 39 of these 50 patients were taking over 20 units of insulin per day. At the end, there were still 39 of them taking more than 20 units of insulin per day.

Another study was done by two German physicians, Wolf and Priess in 1956.[67] In this study, Wolf and Priess placed 60 diabetic patients of all ages and both sexes on a diet containing almost no fat. The diet essentially consisted of rice, potatoes, and fruit. In a matter of only 18 days, the urine in 22 of the patients became completely free of sugar, and the blood-sugar levels in all 60 patients dropped dramatically.

Other more recent studies have been done with similar success. In this country, W. E. Conner had experimented with low-fat dietary treatment of diabetics in the early 1960s and found that patients fared far better on low-fat diets than on other diabetes-control regimens.[62]

In addition to the supporting evidence of direct studies such as those done by Rabinowitch, Wolf-Priess, and Conner, there was also plenty of indirect evidence from studies of primitive populations that supported the low-fat diet as a means of preventing diabetes. The Papuan people of New Guinea are typical of the primitive population groups that have been studied. Luyken and his associates studied in some detail the nutritional habits of a group of more than 21,000 Papuans.[56] This group of people subsists almost wholly on the sweet potato and its leaves. An analysis of this diet showed that it contains only 3 percent fat; the bulk of the diet, 94 percent, is complex carbohydrates and the remainder, 3 per cent, protein. A group of 777 adults was tested, and not one case of diabetes was found. Not only that, but their glucose tolerance responses (a measure of a person's bent toward diabetes) remained normal across all age groups. This can be compared with high-fat diets in Western cultures in which glucose tolerance responses are increasingly diabetic with increasingly older groups.

Of course it could be argued, and it was in fact argued for some years, that there are genetic reasons why some populations are prone to diabetes while others seem not to be. However, the concept of a genetic origin for diabetes has been hard to square with what is known about the disease and its occurrence in different races. African Bantu natives, for example, are free of diabetes, and their blood fats and blood-sugar levels are normally very low. It might be thought that these low blood-sugar levels are caused by the Bantu's genes, and that in some way these same genes protect the Bantu from diabetes. Yet in a study of Bantu prisoners who were fed a diet similar to a normal American diet (namely, high in fats), it was found that their blood fats and blood-sugar responses quickly shifted in the direction of the diabetic.[36] Soon their blood-sugar levels and blood-fat levels matched those levels common in America and in other Western cultures. Clearly it is the Bantu diet that causes these low blood-sugar levels—not Bantu genes.

Observations such as these with the Bantu, together with the fact that diabetics can be managed by a radical low-fat diet, undermined the notion of diabetes' genetic origins. The fact that there exists a familial pattern to diabetes (that is, that people in a diabetic's family are more likely to be diabetic themselves) could be seen to be completely consistent with the high-fat origins of diabetes, since people in the family of a person with a high-fat diet are more likely to be eating a high-fat diet themselves.

In the light of what is now known, the low-fat diet

emerges as the proper means by which to prevent and control diabetes in most cases, and the genetic-defect concept of diabetes is relegated, at least for most people, to the obscurity of a disproved theory.

It should be pointed out that dietary management of diabetes was tried often in the past, but except for the studies of Rabinowitch, Wolf-Priess, Conner, and a few others, such diets were generally very high in fats, and a very low-fat diet was carefully avoided. The reason for this is due to an ironic technicality. The three main ingredients of any diet are fats, protein, and carbohydrates. To stay alive you need a certain amount of calories, which you can get from any one of these three ingredients. However, you can only get so many of your calories in proteins before you begin to develop serious problems from excess protein intake. Therefore, to eat a very low-fat diet, you wind up needing a very high amount of carbohydrates in your diet. The technicality that prevented researchers from trying high-carbohydrate diets with diabetic people was the following: All carbohydrates are made up of combinations of sugar molecules. When you eat carbohydrates, no matter what kind they are, your body soon breaks them down into sugar molecules. It just did not seem reasonable to most researchers that a diabetic, a person who already has trouble with his sugar levels and, in fact, might pass into a diabetic coma if he were to eat sugar, should be given a diet consisting of nothing more than large complexes of sugar molecules. No high-carbohydrate dietary management (and therefore no low-fat dietary management) of diabetes was thus generally encouraged. In fact, all dietary management of diabetes revolved around diets low in carbohydrates and therefore high in fats.

But there is a world of difference between how the body handles large complexes of sugar molecules (that is, complex carbohydrates) and its handling of sugar all by itself.

As stated above, a carbohydrate molecule is nothing other than a group of sugar molecules. Some carbohydrate molecules are gigantic, literally comprised of thousands of sugar molecules. On the other hand, some carbohydrate molecules are very small, consisting of only a few sugar molecules. Sucrose, for example, is a carbohydrate molecule consisting of only two sugar molecules, a glucose molecule (blood sugar) tied to a fructose molecule (fruit sugar). Sucrose is what you find on the kitchen table—what we ordinarily refer to as "table sugar."

Carbohydrate molecules consisting of only one, two, or a very few sugar molecules are called *simple* carbohydrates. Table sugar, honey, molasses, and syrup are all examples of simple carbohydrates. All the other carbohydrates are called *complex* carbohydrates and typically are made up of very, very large molecules. Complex carbohydrate foods are such things as potatoes, bread (without sugar as an ingredient), corn, spaghetti, and rice.

Simple carbohydrates in the diet convert to fats; they increase blood fats and certain diabetic symptoms. On the other hand, complex carbohydrates have just the opposite effect. In 1966, J. J. Groen and his associates in Israel showed that a diet the carbohydrates of which consisted of simple carbohydrates caused the cholesterol levels in the body to increase very quickly and, in addition, caused the person on such a diet to exhibit definite diabetic symptoms.[33,34] On the other hand, a diet identical in every respect, except that the carbohydrates were complex instead of simple, showed neither of these effects. Other researchers subsequently showed that simple carbohydrate diets produced significantly higher levels of insulin in the blood. Finally, W. W. Shieve of Brookhaven National Laboratory showed in 1971 that subjects on a simple carbohydrate diet for a week to ten days exhibited two to five times as strong a tendency to convert any sugar eaten directly into blood fats as nondiabetics.

A diet of simple carbohydrates thus increases the level of both fats and cholesterol in the blood, and worsens glucose response, whereas a diet of complex carbohydrates does the opposite. Therefore, early researchers' fears that the high-carbohydrate diet would worsen the diabetic's condition were unwarranted (provided such a diet employed complex carbohydrates rather than simple carbohydrates).

The role of simple carbohydrates in the cause of diabetes (and in atherosclerosis) is an example of the sensitivity of the human organism to diet. Simple carbohydrates are what the human ultimately needs to obtain the energy required to run the body's cellular machinery. Yet our bodies have apparently evolved over some millions of years to derive these simple carbohydrates not directly from simple carbohydrates but rather from complex carbohydrates. Perhaps the reason for this is that free, simple carbohydrates are relatively rare in nature, honey being the best example. Complex carbohydrates such as those found in grain, roots, and leaves (or simple carbohydrates locked into other material like the fructose bound up in fruit), on the other hand, are abundant; to survive, we must have had to get most of our energy requirements from them.

When we put a complex carbohydrate (say, a bite of potato) into our stomach, our body immediately sets out to break it down into its component simple sugars. Over a period of hours, the bite of potato is broken down into its simple sugar components, and thus the sugar components of the potato trickle into our bloodstream a little at a time. Insulin levels and fat levels in the blood that result from this slow trickle are exactly what our body needs (and for which it clearly has been evolutionarily designed).

But when we eat free, simple carbohydrates (say, a candy bar), simple sugars pour into our bloodstream in a torrent, and in a few minutes the entire sugar content of the candy bar has made its way into the blood. The result is that the insulin level goes way too high along with the fat level.

This high level of insulin causes sugar to be burned rapidly, bringing the blood-sugar level down once again. But due to the high initial level of insulin, the blood sugar usually drops lower than normal, resulting in disturbing symptoms of hypoglycemia (low blood sugar). You may have noticed such symptoms in yourself, if you have ever skipped lunch and instead had a candy bar and a cup of coffee. The dizziness and weakness that you may have experienced later on in the afternoon, after such a "lunch," is likely to be caused simply by sugar-induced hypoglycemia.

Paradoxically, eating sugar thus leads to subsequent low-sugar levels in the blood for the normal person. Not only does the candy bar lead to a state of hypoglycemia, it also leads to a state of higher blood fats, as already noted. Although an elevation in blood fats does not always immediately produce the symptoms that are associated with hypoglycemia, it is nevertheless an undesirable condition to maintain chronically because of its known role in both diabetes and atherosclerosis.

Free, simple carbohydrates taken as food simply give the body too much of a good thing too quickly, even though the body eventually needs simple carbohydrates.

Diabetes is like atherosclerosis. Its prevention and treatment can be effected, not by drugs, but by diet. It is interesting to see that dietary fat, an important culprit in atherosclerosis, is also an important culprit in diabetes. It is also interesting to see that sugars have a role in both atherosclerosis and diabetes because of their ability to raise blood fats and cholesterol. At this point, it would not be surprising to find that these diseases are in some way related to each other, over and above the fact that they are brought on by the same dietary elements. And in fact there is a strong connection between diabetes and atherosclerosis. The diabetic is many times more prone to death and disability due to atherosclerosis than is the nondiabetic.[68] In addition, it is well known that men who are hospitalized with an acute myocardial infarction—the most common result of atherosclerosis and the most common type of heart attack—will often show a diabetic response to a glucose tolerance test. There is thus a clear connection, albeit not entirely understood, between the incidence of diabetes and atherosclerosis and heart disease, just as there is a connection between the dietary elements that cause them.

To summarize, individuals with diabetes who have been treated with insulin injections have historically had a poor long-term prognosis: blindness, heart disease, gangrene, and so forth. Furthermore, one of the fundamental reasons for giving insulin injections to all diabetics disappeared when it was discovered that the diabetic's pancreas was often not only capable of self-generating insulin, but indeed often generated more insulin than that of the nondiabetic. With the discoveries about the diabetic's pancreas and the role of blood fats in causing diabetic symptoms, the notion of the low-fat diet for controlling diabetes was born. Experience with low-fat diets and evidence of the lack of diabetes in primitive groups of people who have essentially low-fat diets have brought forth the low-fat, high-carbohydrate diet as the only viable means for preventing and treating diabetes in most cases. The carbohydrates in such a diet must of necessity exclude the simple carbohydrates: table sugar, honey, molasses, and so forth, which have the property of increasing blood fats and increasing the clinical signs of diabetes. Diabetes and atherosclerosis are related: They are caused by certain of the same dietary elements and, in addition, a person who has diabetes is very likely to develop atherosclerosis and vice versa.

A Backward Look at Some of Our Mistakes with Diabetes
We cannot get away from the fact that for 50 years diabetes

was thought to be caused exclusively by a defective pancreas. This and other mistaken ideas inevitably led to confusion, incorrect notions, and plain bad treatment. It is important that we look back over some of the mistakes that have been made, because there still exists a good deal of confusion, and some mistakes are still being practiced. You should be aware of the main points of confusion.

Although insulin was considered the miracle breakthrough 50 years ago, its complications—blindness, heart disease, and so forth—tarnished the insulin image. In addition, it became known in modern years that injected insulin has a way of seriously damaging the pancreas and the body's own insulin-producing capacity, so that once started on it, a diabetic often had to continue using it despite its dangers. A person who was thus mistakenly diagnosed as a diabetic and received insulin injections was often irreparably turned into a diabetic by the treatment itself.

Diabetes has also been inadvertently "caused" in other ways. It turns out, for example, that a person who has to spend upwards of 10 days in bed because of injury or illness often shows blood-sugar responses indicating diabetes. But in fact the person is not diabetic at all, and all his responses return to normal as soon as he resumes his customary activities. However, if an overzealous physician incorrectly decides that his patient is diabetic and puts him on insulin, his life may be tragically ruined from that point onward.

In the 1940s and early 1950s insulin was used as a shock therapy for schizophrenics. Tremendous doses of insulin were given to induce insulin coma and certain types of convulsions. This drastic therapy not only created diabetics out of its recipients, but also increased the incidence of coma-induced brain damage as well.

The long and short of it was that insulin lost its glamor, and when oral drugs for controlling blood-sugar levels in diabetics came out in the late 1950s, they were welcomed

How to Solve the Problem 61

with much relief by the medical community. Drugs could be taken orally instead of by injection, and thus were much more convenient to the user. The drugs were subjected to extensive testing before being put to general use, and when finally introduced were enthusiastically and widely accepted. But the problem of diabetic complications continued.

As years passed, much discussion among physicians and researchers concerning the relative merits of oral drugs, insulin, and diet control took place. In order to decide which was the superior treatment producing the least complications, a large-scale experiment was devised. The experiment [37] entitled the University Group Diabetes Program (UGDP), funded by a Federal grant, was conducted by 50 scientists and involved 12 hospitals in the United States and Puerto Rico. Taking part were over 1,000 patients, who were all placed on the same diet and divided into four equal groups. Group 1 was on diet alone. The conventional high-fat diet—20 percent protein, 40 percent fat—that had been used for years, was modified to 35 percent fat. Group 2 was on diet plus a popular oral drug, Orinase. Groups 3 and 4 were on diet and insulin, with the insulin used in both fixed and variable doses to test some popular dosage ideas. A fifth group was added a year later to the general program. The patients in this group used the same diet plus a newer oral drug, Phenformin.

The study was carefully designed to prevent any sort of accidental bias arising from the study results. The Group 1 patients on diet alone took a sugar tablet or capsule which was identical in appearance to the Orinase and Phenformin capsules. Even the physicians treating the patients for the entire study did not know who was on the sugar tablet until the first results were announced.

The announcement of the study results was greeted with wild disbelief and dismay by many. Angry fights among study physicians and many nonstudy physicians were reported in medical publications. But regardless of the opinions held, all were stunned by the results, which included:

1. Orinase plus diet resulted in 250 percent more atherosclerosis-related deaths than diet alone.
2. Phenformin plus diet resulted in 250 percent more atherosclerosis-related deaths than diet alone.
3. Insulin, either in fixed or variable dose, resulted in the same number of atherosclerosis-related deaths as diet alone.
4. On the diabetic diet alone there were more atherosclerosis-related deaths in diabetics than in nondiabetics.

The study also brought out some revealing observations:

1. Control of diabetes by oral drugs or insulin does not prevent or delay the appearance of complications.
2. It is possible that asymptomatic patients would fare better if they were not diagnosed as diabetic and not treated as diabetics.

As a result of the UGDP findings the Food and Drug Administration (FDA) issued a statement agreeing with the conclusions and proposing that the oral drugs not be used. This proposal was not well received by some physicians in the largest diabetic clinics. For example, 40 of the nation's leading diabetologists, under the leadership of the medical director of Boston's Joslin Clinic, called upon the FDA to rescind its recommendation. The head of the UGDP study replied: "There is no reason to use these agents until they have been shown to do more good than harm. . . . Lowering blood sugar does not prevent the complications of diabetes. This is the core of the study." [39]

It is interesting to note that the manufacturer of one oral drug said in defense of his product: "There is no question of the effectiveness . . . in lowering the blood sugar of selected patients with diabetes." (Of course no one had questioned that fact. The manufacturer merely neglected to mention that in addition his product was responsible for producing excess deaths.)

In reviewing the results of the study, an American Medical Association spokesman said: "It should not be overlooked that the very best control of blood sugar by experts did not significantly benefit this group of diabetic patients. . . . One might even raise the question of whether physicians should expend time and money to diagnose asymptomatic adult-onset diabetes, if its medical management leads to no significant benefit. If traditional and highly regarded therapy for adult-onset diabetes has no scientific basis and results in no benefit to the patient, it will not be the first cherished therapy to be abandoned. One has only to reflect on the current attitude toward bed rest for the treatment of tuberculosis and to recall how many millions of dollars, staff effort, and patient years were wasted on bed-rest therapy before comparative clinical trials showed it to be of no significant benefit." [105]

The furor over the UGDP results is still going on. It is always difficult to accept and deal with mistakes that have been practiced for years. But these mistakes, like the notion that high unsaturated fat diets will prevent and cure atherosclerosis, will soon become past history. Diabetes is caused by excessively high blood fat levels and its cure and prevention are to be found in reducing these levels by a low-fat, high-carbohydrate (complex only) diet. The book's authors are confident that such a diet for diabetes (and other degenerative diseases) will ultimately gain wide acceptance and usage.

HYPERTENSION

Hypertension Means High Blood Pressure

Hypertension is the condition of having high blood pressure. Hypertension is not a condition of being "very tense" or "very nervous," although the layman often associates the word hypertension with the notion of nervousness or tenseness. Recently the Longevity Foundation did an informal telephone survey in the Boston area to determine what a random sample of individuals thought hypertension means. Although the older age groups appeared to be more likely to know what hypertension means than the younger age groups, it is interesting that more than 60 percent of the people polled did not know the meaning of hypertension. Respondents thought it might mean anything from a state of excitability to a state of edginess. Less than 40 percent of the respondents thought that it meant a state of high blood pressure. Even among those people who knew that hypertension means high blood pressure, a majority felt that this high blood pressure was caused by a state of nerves or tenseness.

However, hypertension has nothing to do with nerves or tenseness. It does not mean nervousness or tenseness, and it is not caused by those conditions. It means simply long-term, continuing high blood pressure, and it is caused by very real physical happenings within the body.

Blood Pressure Standards

Blood in the arteries is always maintained under a certain amount of pressure to insure that all parts of the body receive their necessary supplies of blood, just as tap water in the house is normally under a certain amount of water pressure so that on demand water can be supplied throughout the house. But unlike domestic water pressure, arterial blood pressure is not maintained at a fixed pressure level. Instead, the arterial blood pressure pulses with each beat of the heart to a higher pressure and then back to a lower pressure. Blood pressure is therefore constantly alternating from its peak value to its low value and back again, each time the heart beats. When we talk about an individual's blood pressure then, we cannot talk about a constant value; we need to talk about both the peak value and the low value. A person's blood pressure is thus not a single number; it is a pair of numbers, and this pair of numbers is usually written on paper with the peak pressure first. A blood pressure of 120/70 means that the peak pressure [*] is 120, the low pressure 70.

High blood pressure means that either the peak pressure is higher than it should be, the low pressure is not as low as it should be, or more often that both of these things are true. While 120/70 is thus completely normal, a pressure such as 250/150 is completely abnormal and would be considered by any doctor as high blood pressure. There are persons with blood pressure readings higher than 250/150, and there are individuals with blood-pressure readings lower than 120/70. There are also persons at every possible point in between. The cutoff point that divides hypertension from normal blood pressure is thus somewhat arbitrary. Opinion is divided. Some authorities feel that anything over 140/90 is abnormal, but others feel that blood pressure is only abnormal if it is more than 160/95. In a study of 4 million Americans conducted in 1959 by the Society of Actuaries, entitled "Build and Blood Pressure Study," it was reported that for all ages blood pressures exceeding 140/90 are correlated with excess deaths. Perhaps then the lower figure 140/90 is indeed a reasonable limit for the normal range of blood

---

[*] Pressure is measured in millimeters of mercury.

pressure, since blood pressures above it seem to jeopardize one's life span.

Shifts in Blood Pressure

So far we have talked as if blood pressure is a fixed value, say 120/70, and does not change from that value. But in fact blood pressure is not fixed at any given point, but continuously changes as the demands on the body change. Over a given 24-hour period a person will normally show definite swings in his blood pressure. Also, during physical exertion, a person's blood pressure will rise sharply.[84] For example, systolic pressure (the larger of the two numbers in a blood pressure measurement), during weight lifting, may jump above 250 within a matter of seconds. Long-distance runners may maintain systolic pressure above 180 for hours at a time. These higher pressures during physical exertion are needed to meet the extra requirements of the at-work muscles. Blood pressure is also increased during moments of emotional stress. For example, the adrenalin pumped into the bloodstream at times of acute emotional crisis causes, among other reactions, a sharp increase in blood pressure.

Jumps from time to time in blood pressure are thus normal for the body and are needed to meet the normal demands of living. Furthermore, the body evidently has a definite control system that is used to regulate the body's blood pressure to meet bodily needs. At the writing of this book, the blood pressure control system is not completely understood. We know, however, that it is a complicated system involving certain hormones, the autonomic nervous system, the kidneys, and the electrolyte balance of the blood. But we do not know the details of how it works. Yet we do know that this control system can be thrown out of tolerance in a number of different ways, and once it is out, it is sometimes difficult to bring back to normal. Hypertension is the result of the blood pressure control system getting out of tolerance, and hypertensive disease is the result of leaving it out of tolerance for a long period of time.

Since temporary high blood pressures are a common occurrence on a now-and-then basis anyway, we would not be worried about hypertension if it were not for the disease that can result from it as a sustained condition. If left unchecked, high blood pressure all by itself will often lead to irreversible damage to the thousands of little arteries or arterioles that branch off the main arteries. The brunt of the damage is borne by the little arteries in the kidneys, the pancreas, and the retina of the eye, causing damage and failure in these organs. Hypertension all by itself can thus lead to severe illness and death. This sort of disease condition is often called malignant hypertensive disease.*

In addition, hypertension together with atherosclerosis can cause aneurysms ("blowouts") in the arteries that circulate blood in the brain. Such a blowout is called a cerebral hemorrhage and is a common kind of "stroke" that individuals suffer. Of all the things that can be directly caused by hypertension, cerebral hemorrhage may be the most common and the most dangerous. It makes sense that high blood pressure should threaten to cause arterial blowouts in the same way that over-pressurized automobile tires threaten to cause tire blowouts. But, in fact, it appears that arterial blowouts are unlikely, unless the artery has already been greatly weakened. In experiments with healthy arteries [85] it was thus found that pressures in the several thousands of millimeters of mercury could be withstood by the arteries without bursting. On the other hand, tens of thousands of Americans are stricken every year with cerebral hemorrhage stemming from arteries that have burst under pressures which we may reasonably presume to be at most only

---

* The word malignant here means "severe," not "cancerous" as is commonly thought.

a few hundreds of millimeters of mercury. From what we have already learned about the great extent to which atherosclerosis exists in nearly every person in this country and the arterial fragility that atherosclerosis brings with it, it is no surprise that pressures of only a few hundreds can exceed the strength of the artery and cause it to rupture, producing so many deaths as a result.

The Causes of Hypertension

Hypertension is evidently very common in the United States. In a recent analysis of 22,929 male and female workers in Chicago, Schoenberger and his associates found that nearly one in eight of the people examined were hypertensive.[86] If these statistics are applicable to the entire country, this means that literally millions of Americans are living with the dangers of high blood pressure.

At present there is no agreement among medical researchers and practitioners on the causes of most of these cases of high blood pressure. To be sure, we know the causes of hypertension in many specific cases. We know, for example, that hypertension can be caused by any of the following three things:

1. Atherosclerosis;
2. Excess salt intake;
3. Specific diseases of the kidneys, the adrenals, and the arteries.

But it is not clear to most researchers why such vast numbers of people are afflicted. It is generally believed in the medical community that hypertension is caused either by an increase in the blood output of the heart on each beat or by an increase in the resistance to the blood in the body's arterial system.[87]

Atherosclerosis and Hypertension

It has been known for some time that atherosclerosis can lead in a direct, causal way to high blood pressure by producing plaques in the arteries in the kidney. In addition, actual measurements of the amount of atherosclerosis present in the body shows that the degree of atherosclerosis throughout the body is statistically related to the amount of high blood pressure a person experiences.[88] Furthermore, population studies reveal that population groups who do not have atherosclerosis also do not have hypertension. This is well illustrated by the New Zealand aborigines discussed earlier,[13] who not only are free of heart disease and atherosclerosis but are also free of any hint of hypertension. Their blood pressures begin at low values and remain so throughout their lives. We might compare this with Americans whose average blood pressure levels rise over the years in keeping with their rising levels of atherosclerosis. In fact, the rise in blood pressure is large enough that the "normality" standards used by physicians have to be continually raised as the American ages.[89]

The fact that there is a mechanism for explaining how atherosclerosis can cause hypertension—obstruction of arteries with plaques—together with the fact that, worldwide, there is a convincing association of atherosclerosis with hypertension leads one to believe that atherosclerosis may play more than a minor role in the cause of hypertension. Indeed, as with heart disease, atherosclerosis may cause most of the hypertension that we see. In any case, regardless of the size of the role it plays, it is clear that atherosclerosis does cause considerable hypertension; thus its eradication by the dietary measures discussed earlier will also eradicate much of the hypertension now present in the country.

Salt Intake and Hypertension

Since the late 1940s it has been known that salt in the diet can aggravate human hypertension.[90] Moreover, it was soon discovered that a very low salt diet can reduce hypertension.[91] Many experiments with people and with animals have followed these early discoveries, and it has been shown under a variety of conditions how ordinary salt can produce hypertension and, furthermore, how under some circumstances the resulting hypertension is permanent. That is, it does not go away when salt is once again removed from the diet.

It is unclear at this time exactly how salt achieves its ability to cause hypertension. This is particularly true for the mechanism that causes the blood pressure to remain permanently fixed at a higher level than before. But there is no question that salt does indeed have this property.

In northern Japan extremely high salt intakes are common: an average of nearly an ounce of salt per day per person. This is nearly three times the average in Western urban-oriented cultures such as ours.[92] Not surprisingly, the incidence of hypertension in this northern part of Japan is probably the highest known, approximately 40 percent of the adult population. Furthermore the rate of deaths attributable to hypertensive complications is extremely high, probably higher in this part of Japan than anywhere else in the world.

On the other hand there is a very low incidence of hypertension in several divergent ethnic groups: Greenland Eskimos, aboriginal tribes in the mountains of China, Cuna Indians of Panama, and aboriginal Australians.[92] L. K. Dahl has suggested that this low incidence of hypertension results from a very low intake of salt,[93] less than a fifth of that consumed in Western cultures such as ours.

These and many other similar studies show clearly that

there is a strong presumption that dietary salt has a significant and independent role in the cause of hypertension.

Specific Diseases and Hypertension

Aside from atherosclerosis and salt, there are a number of specific diseases that will cause hypertension. According to current medical beliefs, all diseases that cause hypertension involve the kidneys, and practically all kidney diseases are associated with hypertension.[87] Specific diseases that will cause hypertension range from tumors on the ovaries to diabetic kidney disease. Considering the large number of specific diseases that do cause hypertension, it is interesting to note that according to authoritative estimates only about a third of all cases of hypertension are brought about by all of these specific diseases put together. The other two-thirds are caused by atherosclerosis, salt, or other "unknown" factors.

Treating Hypertension

For years hypertension was treated with low salt diets. And experience has told us that diets that are very low in salt * are effective at bringing high blood pressure under control. However, for acute "malignant" hypertension it sometimes is the case that either it is not possible to bring blood pressure under control or it is not possible to do so fast enough. In cases of very high blood pressure it is desirable to bring blood pressure down immediately, because time lost waiting for dietary measures to take hold can be fatal. The advent of antihypertensive drugs that can bring blood pressure down in a hurry has thus been a big advance in the

---

* Actually it is the sodium in ordinary salt that needs to be limited rather than the specific salt or sodium chloride itself. Therefore antihypertensive diets are really low sodium diets. However, nearly all of our sodium normally comes from ordinary salt. A salt-free diet is thus very nearly a sodium-free diet as well.

field of hypertension. These drugs, which are as good as diet at reducing blood pressure, have been enthusiastically embraced by the medical profession and are now widely being used in place of diet to control hypertension.

However, while there is very good reason to use these drugs for prompt relief of the dangerous cases of malignant hypertension, there is not such good reason to continue using them if dietary measures can be eventually substituted in their place. And there is even less reason to use them for the large majority of hypertension cases in which blood pressure is too high, but not so high as to be imminently life threatening. The reason is that all of the antihypertensive drugs produce side effects. For example, the thiazides are known to elevate uric acid in the blood [94] and to create symptoms of arthritis. Arthritis would hardly be considered a mild side effect. To combat this side effect uricosuric drugs are used with the thiazides. However, they have their own side effects.[95] The two principal drugs of this kind, probenecid and allopurinol, both result in a deposit of crystals in the muscles with the attendant risk of resulting muscle disease. To make things worse, the antihypertensive drugs are lifelong affairs. That is, there is little chance that after even many years on a drug regimen the drugs could be stopped and the blood pressure would remain low. Instead, evidence shows [96] that if the drugs are stopped, the lowered blood pressures also stop: They jump back up to original high values.

To get away from drugs and the ever-present danger of short-term or cumulative side effects, one must switch over to diet sooner or later. From all we know at this time, it appears that the best course of action for anyone to take is not to develop high blood pressure in the first place. The only safe way to do this is with diet rather than drugs, and the diet that will do the most to prevent hypertension has the following features. It is:

1. Salt free;
2. Nonatherogenic* (namely, low fat, low cholesterol, low sugar).

OTHER FACTORS IN THE CAUSES OF DEGENERATIVE DISEASES

In the previous pages we have discussed the primary factors in the cause of the degenerative diseases. Two other factors that play a comparatively smaller but nevertheless an important role in causing such diseases are caffeine and cigarette smoking. Let us take a quick look in this section at these two factors and see what they do.

Cigarette Smoking

So much has been said and written about the adverse effects of cigarette smoking on health that it hardly warrants more elaboration in this book. We shall, however, make a few important observations about tobacco and the degenerative diseases.

People have been concerned about the effects of tobacco on health ever since tobacco was introduced into Western culture by the American Indians back in the times of Columbus. Tobacco has been condemned as harmful to the lungs and other organs since earliest times,[121] even though valid statistical evidence was not available, and such condemnation was apparently based solely on the general appearance and behavior of tobacco users. By 1900, the use of chewing tobacco and pipe tobacco had risen to about 4 pounds and 2½ pounds, respectively, per person, per year in the United States, and cigarette smoking had climbed to about 140 cigarettes per person per year.[122] By 1961

---

* Meaning it does not cause atherosclerosis.

cigarette smoking in the United States had climbed to nearly 4,000 cigarettes per person anually.

And in all this time, deaths from heart disease, lung cancer, emphysema, and other diseases have steadily risen. Despite the long-standing belief among laymen and professionals alike that cigarette smoking was harmful to health, it was not until 1964 that the Surgeon General brought forth the classic report *Smoking and Health* (Public Health Service Publication Number 1103). Once and for all it demonstrated with convincing statistical validity that cigarette smoking causes many thousands of deaths every year. Since that time cigarette advertisements have been banned from commercial television, and all cigarette packages have been required to bear the now familiar admonition:

Warning: The Surgeon General Has Determined That Cigarette Smoking Is Dangerous to Your Health

In cigarette smokers, death from lung cancer is more than 1,000 percent higher than it is for nonsmokers.[123] The statistics for heart disease are not nearly so dramatic: In cigarette smokers, death from heart disease (coronaries) is only 70 percent higher than it is for nonsmokers. However, because so many more people die of heart disease than of lung cancer, it turns out that the heart disease deaths that are apparently caused by cigarettes are far greater than the lung cancer deaths caused by cigarettes.[124]

Cigarettes thus appear to do their most damage each year in the area of heart disease. Two other degenerative diseases are also related to cigarette smoking. Both atherosclerosis and hypertension deaths are 50 percent higher among cigarette smokers than nonsmokers.[123]

Abstinence from cigarette smoking is therefore important from the point of view of avoiding death or disability from heart disease or from the degenerative diseases as a whole. But even aside from the degenerative diseases, cigarette smoking is so deleterious to health—in so many different ways—that its avoidance is an absolute must to good health. It should also be noted that for people who have stopped smoking, even though they may have smoked for a long time, the probability of death from all causes is substantially less than those who continue to smoke.[125]

Caffeine

We tend to think of coffee and tea as safe beverages; in fact, practically all diets permit the drinking of black coffee or tea with no restriction whatever. However, there is growing and convincing evidence that the caffeine in coffee and tea may be an important factor in the cause of the degenerative diseases.

In 1963, O. Paul reported in a study of heart disease in approximately 2,000 Western Electric employees in Chicago that the frequency of heart disease was positively and significantly related to the amount of coffee consumed.[126] This came as a surprise to many people in the field of heart disease research, but since Paul's group was statistically small, some doubt remained as to the causal nature of the relationship between heart disease and coffee.

Later, Oscar Jankelson and his co-workers showed that coffee had the direct effect of altering the human glucose response curves so that individuals showed up as "more diabetic" after drinking coffee than before.[127] This caused Jankelson and his associates some apprehension, and they called for large-scale investigations to study these "adverse effects" of coffee.

Although large-scale investigations have not come about, other important pieces of clinical evidence have been acquired. In 1968, Samuel Bellet showed that coffee drinking increases the free fatty acid levels in the blood.[128] With our knowledge of the role that blood fats cause in atherosclerosis and the other degenerative diseases, it immediately becomes clear how coffee drinking could increase the incidence of heart disease (as shown by Paul). Later, in 1972, Bellet showed that the caffeine in coffee also can lead directly to conditions predisposing to the fibrillation type of heart attack.[129] With dogs he showed that the ventricular fibrillation threshold was decreased after the dogs had been administered caffeine. In essence, caffeine made it easier for Bellet and his co-workers to cause fibrillations in the hearts of the experimental dogs.

In short, coffee (and in particular the caffeine in coffee) appears to increase the incidence of heart disease. The mechanisms for how this might be brought about are partly known, and they imply that caffeine may also increase the incidence of other degenerative diseases as well. To these effects of caffeine must be added the fact that it may have a role in the production of cancer. Kuhlman and his associates have shown that caffeine causes chromatid breakage in human cells, like the breakage that occurs when a person is exposed to radiation. In fact, they estimate that one cup of coffee is equivalent to .01 roentgens of radiation * exposure in the X band. In their own words: "There is a strong likelihood that caffeine may prove to be one of the most dangerous mutagens in man." [130]

The warnings are clear: Caffeine is likely to be dangerous to health. The authors therefore believe that coffee, tea, and other substances containing caffeine should be avoided.

---

* Four to five hundred roentgens of absorbed radiation is almost always fatal if over a short period of time (minutes or hours). Over a lifetime absorbed radiation can be higher than this without fatality. How much higher depends on the person and on the type of radiation. In the case of caffeine, which is not radiation, but which acts in its mutagenesis like radiation, no fatality estimates can be made without further data.

CHAPTER 3

The Role of Exercise

It is very clear to most people today that regular physical exercise is an important part of good health. Physical exercise can give the average person extra strength, endurance, and coordination, not to mention improved appearance, posture, and mental outlook. The President's Council on Physical Fitness, in its book on adult physical fitness, points out that exercise can eliminate chronic tiredness, tension, and minor body pains. In addition, it is known that exercise aids in controlling overweight and maintaining health during old age.

As if all these benefits of exercise were not quite enough, it turns out that exercise plays an important role in the prevention and reversal of degenerative diseases as well. Each of the degenerative diseases can be reduced in severity by proper exercise alone, although as we discussed in the last chapter, attention to the sort of food we eat is an essential prerequisite. In this chapter we are going to go over the effects of exercise on the three specific degenerative diseases discussed in the last chapter: heart disease, diabetes, and hypertension. Exercise is a vital part of the 2100 Program, and when you see how it affects these diseases, you will know why.

Exercise and Heart Disease

Many studies over the years seem to show that exercise can protect us, at least partly, from heart disease. In 1958, Paul Dudley White and William C. Pomeroy completed an interesting study of 335 former athletes whose athletic careers were primarily in the time period 1901 to 1930.[40] It was found that none of the men studied who maintained a heavy exercise regimen after retiring from sports suffered a heart attack. On the other hand, about a third of the other athletes analyzed had died from a heart attack.

In 1962, Taylor and his workers studied the health records of more than 20,000 railroad employees and classified deaths from heart disease according to the employees' type of work.[41] Taylor found that twice as many railroad clerks died of heart disease as the more active railroad switchmen.

The famous Framingham study that began in 1948 and continued through 1971 showed that the death rate from heart disease was five times as great for the most inactive men as for the most active men in the study.[42] In 1968, Kidera reported in the *Journal of the American Medical Association* that exercise can convert an abnormal electrocardiogram (EKG) to normal.[43]

All these studies and many more convinced most people that exercise was important in protecting against heart disease. Its protection apparently derives from its ability to get around the effects of atherosclerosis.

Atherosclerosis causes heart disease by clogging the coronary arteries, the small arteries that nourish the heart muscle. When all the coronary arteries are clean and open, the entire heart muscle receives the blood it needs to pump properly. Under these conditions the heart muscle takes on a healthy pink color. But when some of this blood supply is reduced, the part of the heart that is affected will become starved for oxygen and develop a bluish color. A diseased heart might be receiving plenty of oxygen and be pink in one area while being blue and starved for oxygen in other areas. Where a blue area and a pink area meet, a line forms, called an *oxygen differential* line. There is a large difference in the amount of oxygen reaching the heart on one side of this line over that reaching the heart on the other.

As far back as 1955 Claude Beck and David Leighninger in Cleveland discovered [117] that these oxygen differentials were responsible for a great many heart disease deaths. They found that an evenly oxygenated heart—whether poorly oxygenated or well oxygenated—is very unlikely to fail. If the heart thus is all pink or all blue, failure is unlikely. (Of course, if it stays blue, the entire heart muscle may eventually die from oxygen starvation.) But a heart checkerboarded with areas of blue and pink, indicating many lines of oxygen differentials, is very likely to fail.

Beck and Leighninger found that oxygen differential lines cause the heart muscle to contract better on the high side of the line than on its low side, which in turn may cause the heart muscle to be thrown into a spasm of fluttering or uncoordinated trembling instead of a strong, coordinated beating rhythm. This very common sort of heart attack is called a fibrillation.

After the work by Beck and Leighninger, it became clear why so many people died under conditions of sudden physical exertion. Many persons have coronary arteries that are partly blocked by atherosclerosis disease, so that their heart muscles receive uneven supplies of blood in the muscles' various parts. The received oxygen supply may be adequate so that a person's heart is completely pink as long as he is relatively at rest. But if he finds himself strenuously shoveling snow one day, the demand for blood to his heart may jump so much that the uneven blood supply begins to show itself by creating the blue and pink oxygen differentials which will cause a sudden heart attack.

At first glance this seems like quite a problem. We know that exercise can protect us from heart disease, yet there are many cases in which sudden and heavy exercise can cause quick death from heart attack. The answer to this problem is, of course, that any exercise program has to start easy and build strength gradually. Too much exercise too soon in a person with atherosclerosis (which is nearly all of us) can be a very dangerous thing indeed.

What happens when we exercise over a long time is that additional routes of blood supply are built up in the heart. The coronary arteries grow in size, and the places where the arteries are blocked grow new routes for carrying blood.[44,45,46,47] These new routes of blood have the effect of keeping the heart thoroughly oxygenated (thoroughly pink), even under hard exercise. But to obtain new growth takes time and patience. It takes a program of exercise which gets harder only on a gradual basis. Any attempt to hurry the process up can be as dangerous as Russian roulette. It should be pointed out that exercise does not unclog the arteries. It simply helps to make new paths around the clogs. Only care in what we eat can unclog the arteries by shrinking arterial atherosclerotic plaques.

Once the heart is healthy again and fully oxygenated, evidence indicates that no amount of exercise will cause the heart to fibrillate. This was well demonstrated in the 1968 Olympics, which were held in Mexico City. Since Mexico City is 7,000 feet above sea level, an unprecedented number of athletes who had trained at lower altitudes collapsed from overexertion.[48] Some of these may even have overexerted so much as to cause their hearts to be starved for oxygen. Yet no cases of fibrillation happened. These athletes' hearts are examples of well-oxygenated hearts, which even under oxygen starvation would turn blue evenly all over with no remaining areas of pink. Oxygen-differential fibrillation thus cannot occur in such hearts.

We have just stated that exercise does not protect against heart disease by reducing the underlying atherosclerosis but simply does its good by getting around the existing atherosclerosis. This definitely seems to be so, yet there is some indirect evidence that atherosclerosis may be partially reversed by exercise. Exercise helps to dissolve a protein in the blood called fibrin.[49,50,51,52,53] Lots of exercise thus means low fibrin levels in the blood. Since blood clots cannot form without fibrin present, it appears that exercise may help to prevent clotting in the blood, which may in turn help to prevent the growth and spread of new atherosclerosis plaques. Exercise thus perhaps stops the spread of atherosclerosis. On the other hand, perhaps it does not. We simply do not know yet.

Exercise and Hypertension

Hypertension (high blood pressure) is also dramatically reduced by exercise alone. In the last chapter we mentioned the fact that, within limits, blood pressure is determined by two things: the amount of blood pumped by the heart per second and the resistance that the blood meets as it courses through the arteries. Exercise has the effect of causing the growth of new capillary arteries and other new routes of blood flow, as previously mentioned. This results in an unavoidable, direct drop in the total resistance of the arterial system.* Even though the ability of the heart to do work

---

* This is true provided that the resistance of the arterial system is not overwhelmingly controlled by a single pathological feature, such as a kidney artery blockage. In that case, resistance would be materially affected only by a removal of the kidney block.

increases with exercise, the net effect of the drop in arterial resistance is to cause a significant decrease in blood pressure.

It has been known for years that in societies where the life style causes people to do a great deal of physical activity, high blood pressure is nearly absent. The primitive Bantu people in southern Africa mentioned earlier are an example. Their life styles require heavy exercise, and their blood pressures show it, remaining low throughout their lives. The Masai in Kenya are also a striking example of this phenomenon. George Mann and his associates in 1964 reported that the Masai have little or no hypertension, and there is virtually none of the increase in blood pressure with age that occurs in all modern industrialized cultures.[106] In describing the Masai in 1965 Mann pointed out [107] that the Masai individual traditionally experienced high levels of physical activities throughout his life.[107] As a child he would tend herds of animals and would cover many miles every day on foot. As an adult he would travel, almost daily, long distances on foot in overseeing his property and herds and visiting with distant friends. An interesting sidelight to the lack of hypertension in these people is the high degree of conditioning obtained. Mann reports that the average Masai male has physical-conditioning levels that match those of champion Olympic athletes.

In addition to the ample amounts of indirect cultural data such as that from the Bantu and the Masai, there also is a substantial and convincing body of direct data on the link between exercise and hypertension. Garret and his coworkers in 1965 found that physical conditioning consistently reduced the diastolic blood pressure in American men.[108] Recently John Hanson and William Nedde at the University of Vermont [109] experimented with a group of men who were already suffering from high blood pressure. For seven months the men were provided with regular physical training involving distance running, calisthenics, and competitive sports. At the end of this time it was found that the average blood pressures of these men at rest had gone from 168/92 down to 134/75. This direct evidence of the beneficial effect of exercise on people who already have hypertensive disease is very important. It tells us that in addition to helping to prevent high blood pressure, exercise also helps to *cure* high blood pressure.

It should be noted that in the Hanson-Nedde study, those patients who fared the best were the ones whose blood pressure was high but still fluctuating (those with labile hypertension). Those whose blood pressure control mechanisms had already become "locked" onto a higher plateau (those with essential hypertension) fared less well. And those whose hypertension was caused by kidney artery blockage (those with organic hypertension) fared least well of all. Exercise thus produced the best effect with those whose hypertension was of lesser severity. However, the evidence indicates that exercise will help high blood pressure at all stages, and the sooner initiated, the better.

Exercise and Diabetes

In the last chapter we learned that diabetes can be caused in normal individuals by feeding them enough fats and simple carbohydrates to raise the levels of fat in their blood. Raised levels of fat, by an unknown mechanism, caused the normally effective insulin in these individuals' blood to lose its effectiveness. With less effective insulin, sugar in the blood cannot be properly used; instead it will build up to high levels.

It is known that when a diabetic exercises, he uses his blood fats for energy rather than stored sugar as a nondiabetic does.[54] With continued exercise, the fat levels in the diabetic's blood are decreased. As they go down his insulin becomes sensitized, and he becomes less diabetic. In 1971, F. J. Buys and his associates in Johannesburg reported their work with eight diabetic patients.[55] Each of the eight individuals completed vigorous exercises for half an hour each day for a period of eight months. At the end of this time symptoms of diabetes had disappeared for seven of the eight patients.

Experiments such as that done by Buys and his co-workers have been conducted by other researchers around the world. It is clear that diabetics are greatly benefited by vigorous exercise. Reversal of diabetes (as in atherosclerosis) must, however, include careful diet as well as regular exercise. To bring blood fats down, the diabetic must permanently lower his intake of fats and simple carbohydrates. Exercise may bring rapid results, but permanent food changes are needed for permanent reversal of diabetes.

CHAPTER 4

The Role of Nutrients

VITAMINS, AMINO ACIDS, MINERALS, CARBOHYDRATES, AND FATS

Although this book deals with nutrition in relation to degenerative diseases, we are going to take a short trip in this chapter into some other details concerning nutrition. This side trip is an absolute must for two reasons. First, it will give a broad picture of the steps a person should take to provide himself with the nutrition needed for good health. In the last few chapters we have emphasized what one should *not* do to avoid degenerative diseases. But there is a lot more to health than "should nots," and this chapter will help to balance those with the "shoulds" of good nutrition.

Second, this chapter is a must because it will provide the intelligent perspective needed to see around the barrage of conflicting and confusing advice one can expect to get from all sides about how vitamins, amino acids, and so forth affect heart disease, diabetes, and the other degenerative diseases. Needless to say much of this advice is erroneous. But, seemingly, everybody has some advice to give about nutrition from the bricklayer to the Nobel prize-winning chemist, and everybody's advice is different. For your own protection it is thus vital that you have some exposure to this chapter's material.

Nutrition: The Big Picture

There are many components of good health, some having to do with mental stress, some with exercise, and some with the food we eat. The subject of nutrition deals only with the food we eat. The only way our bodies can get all the nutrients that are needed to run smoothly is to extract these nutrients from food. For millions of years man has been extracting his nutrients from the food he eats. It is the same today as it has always been, except that today we know a lot more about the nutritional ingredients that are contained in food.

These nutritional ingredients are such substances as vitamins, minerals, amino acids, carbohydrates, and fats. To understand more fully the value of the ingredients in food, there are certain observations we would make. The first observation is that all the nutrients in food are chemicals. Of course, everything in the entire world can be viewed as combinations of chemicals, so this is not a surprising observation. But in particular, the food we eat—any kind of food—is composed of a tremendous variety of chemicals, and it is important for us to recognize that modern nutrition is concerned *only* with what kind of chemicals are needed for good health and how these chemicals work in the body.

The second observation is that our body is a gigantic collection of living cells just as a nation is a collection of living people. These cells are born, and they have a natural life span, just as a country's citizens are born and live out their lives. Our bodies can be healthy if, and *only* if, the cells that comprise them are healthy. What makes a human being healthy is the health of all the trillions of living cells making up his body.

We also need to observe that every single cell in our body is an elaborate, dynamic chemical factory. Each cell takes chemicals into itself, changes its size or shape according to production requirements, and creates chemicals that are shipped out to other cells. Of course, the many kinds of cells—muscle cells, brain cells, blood cells, and so forth—each has its own job to do. A bone cell does not take in the same chemicals as a blood cell; it does not look like a blood cell, and it does not manufacture the same chemicals. But the fact remains that every cell is a complex chemical factory.

From the three observations above, we can glean three fundamental concepts underlying the science of nutrition. These concepts are:

1. Human cells are chemical factories that need to be fed the right chemicals so as to do their jobs.
2. Human beings can be healthy if, and only if, their cells are receiving the right chemicals.
3. The science of nutrition attempts to find out exactly what chemicals are needed by the body cells, and how these chemicals are used.

These fundamental concepts need to be clearly pointed out because they are implicitly contained in all the modern thinking on nutrition.

When we talk about the use of food in our bodies, there are two parts to the picture. The first has to do with identifying the needed chemicals in our food; the second has to do with describing how these chemicals work in the body.

Luckily, in this book we are interested only in the first part of the picture: what chemicals are needed. For even though science is far from knowing all the answers about what is needed, the picture here is far more complete and far simpler than the question of how these chemicals are used. A lot is thus known about what chemicals the body needs, but little is known about the details of how they are used. One reason for this is that the body's needs are relatively simple. The body needs only a few basic ingredients which it gets by breaking down consumed food into component chemicals, keeping what is needed and throwing the rest away. Since the body does not need very much, it has been fairly easy to get some kind of handle on what these needs are.

But imagine how complex the other half of the picture must be. From these few basic ingredients every single item in the body must be manufactured, from blood cells to hormones to skin tissue. An utterly bewildering array of things must be made from these ingredients, and the processes by which this is done remain only vaguely known or guessed at today.

It is thus fortunate, for the sake of a simple discussion, that we only have to consider the chemicals the body needs, not how the body uses these chemicals. Figure 5 opposite shows the six general classes of chemicals that are needed by the body (not including the air we breathe and the water we drink). Notice that one of these classes is called "Unidentified Essential Chemicals." This class was included to show that there is still a lot of ignorance left in the field of nutrition. It is almost certain that there are chemicals essential to good health which have not yet been identified as being essential. The history of nutrition is one long story of finding new things that are vital to health that we did not know about before. In fact, new vitamins are still being discovered.

The six classes of chemicals shown on the right de-

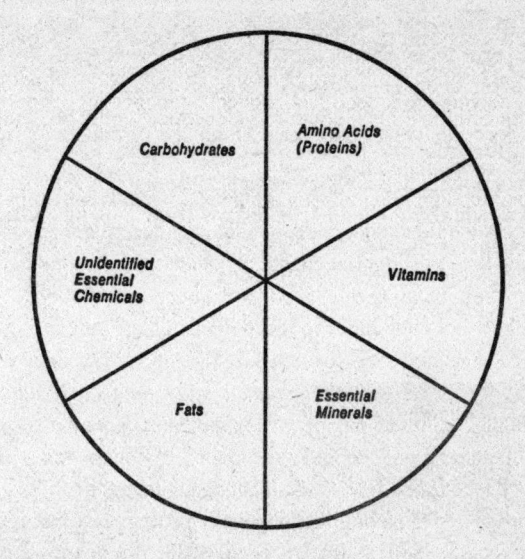

Figure 5. The Six Classes of Chemicals Needed by the Body

fine the types of chemicals needed as food by the body, although one class is admittedly just a place-holder class for those essential chemicals we have yet to discover. We shall discuss each of these six classes below.

Carbohydrates

Inside each body cell there are many chemical processes going on. It is absolutely essential to life that these processes be kept in continuous operation. To keep them going, the cell needs energy just as an automobile factory needs electrical and natural gas energy to keep its equipment running so that the assembly line never stops. The cell can get energy from any one of three of the types of chemicals in the diagram above: from fats, from amino acids (some of them), or from carbohydrates. Of these three sources the cleanest and most direct is carbohydrates, the body's preferred energy source. When carbohydrates are used to generate energy, the cell gets energy with by-products: water and carbon dioxide. This is all, no other waste products. When either fats or amino acids are used, the cell gets energy plus relatively complex waste products which are significantly more difficult to dispose of.

Even though carbohydrates are the preferred energy source, it is a very good thing that the body, if necessary, can use fats and amino acids for energy. In fact, during times when food is plentiful and there are more carbohydrates available than the body needs to use for energy, it will convert some of the carbohydrates to fat and store them away for a rainy day. When that rainy day comes and food is scarce, these fat reserves can be called into play to give the energy needed to keep the cell factories going. And if things remain so bad that all the fat reserves are used up, our bodies can then begin to use body protein as a last resort (muscle, skin, and so forth), breaking it down into amino acids and getting the necessary energy from the amino acids themselves.

Carbohydrates are the trademark of the plant world. More than half of the dry weight of most plants is carbohydrate. Various kinds of carbohydrates are used in every cell in all plants, and they have many roles, the biggest one probably being to act as the plant's walls and structures. So when we eat fruit, vegetables, grain cereals, or any other form of plant life, we are eating carbohydrates. To be sure, we are eating other things besides carbohydrates; nuts, for example, can be as much as 30 per cent fat by weight.

Not all carbohydrates can be used by human beings. The most common of all carbohydrates is cellulose, the carbohydrate that makes up the cell walls of trees, grass, and many other plants. Because our own body cells cannot make an enzyme called cellulase, it turns out that cellulose cannot be broken down in our body for energy. Cows (and many other species) harbor a bacteria that makes cellulose, and can therefore do quite well on a diet of cellulose.

Not all carbohydrates are manufactured by plants. Many of the carbohydrates we eat are manufactured by animals. Lactose, for example, is a simple carbohydrate that along with protein is found in milk. In fact, in cow's milk there is somewhere in the neighborhood of 30 percent more carbohydrate than there is protein. Beef liver, pork liver, and bacon all contain a measurable carbohydrate content, and all animal products contain some carbohydrate molecules, even if only in very small quantities.

Nowadays most of us are taught to think of carbohydrates as "empty calorie" foods—foods that make one fat but not healthy, and foods that we only eat because we are somehow too dumb or too weak-willed to eat food that is "good" for us. We think of the word "starch" (which is a complex carbohydrate built from simple ones) in the same way. Well, carbohydrates and starches deserve another look, because nothing could be further from the truth.

In the first place, one has to understand that there is a great deal of difference between the carbohydrates in a cupcake, and, for example, those that you might get in a plate of lima beans. The carbohydrate in a cupcake is largely the simple sugar, sucrose (plain table sugar). On the other hand, lima beans are largely made up of a carbohydrate which is essentially thousands of sugar molecules tied together in long strings. Carbohydrates that are composed of many sugar molecules put together are called starches. So lima beans are mainly a certain kind of starch.

Let us ask ourselves what we feel is wrong with starches or carbohydrates in our foods. Most people probably would answer that starch and carbohydrates will do two bad things: First, they will give us no vitamins or other nutrients required for health; and second, they will make us fat. Let us think about the question of vitamins and nutrients. In truth, the cupcake will probably provide almost nothing in the way of vitamins and nutrients, as well as being chockfull of fats and sugars (simple carbohydrates). So it makes sense to avoid cupcakes. No problem. But the lima beans are entirely different. A three-ounce serving of lima beans has fewer calories than a one-ounce cupcake, and furthermore, it has 40 milligrams of calcium, 2 milligrams of iron, 225 units of vitamin A, 14 milligrams of vitamin C, and a large assortment of other vitamins and minerals. The lima beans thus have plenty of needed vitamins and nutrients.

But there's still the question of getting too fat. Lima beans and other starches make you fat just as the low-carbohydrate diet books say, right? The answer seems to be no—not if you stick to the lima bean-type carbohydrate. Of course, if you put sugar on your lima beans, butter them, or cook then in fat, that's a different question.

Most people find it difficult to get fat on a diet consisting purely of fruits and vegetables. In Chapter 3 we spoke of the sweet potato eaters in New Guinea,[56] a group of primitive people who throughout their lives eat little more than sweet potatoes and sweet potato leaves. This is a very high carbohydrate diet indeed (94 percent of the food energy comes from carbohydrates). Evidently, sweet potatoes taken together with their leaves contain all the ingredients necessary for life, because these people have healthy lives—and more to the point, they are not fat. It has been the experience of people associated with the Longevity Foundation that it is hard to get fat on a diet consisting of complex starches (like lima beans or other vegetables, grain, etc.), even if one tries hard to do so.

While we are on the subject of carbohydrates making people fat, it is well to amplify a point that we obliquely touched upon in our earlier discussion of diabetes. Lately there has been some concern expressed in the nutrition literature about a phenomenon called *carbohydrate-induced lipemia*. Lipemia is the term used for the condition of having too high a level of fat in the blood. The concern of many nutritionists has revolved around an increase in the fat level of the blood caused by eating carbohydrates. There are many reasons why high-fat levels in the blood are undesirable. We have talked about them in Chapter 3. Thus it is important for us to find out what is behind peoples' concern with respect to carboyhdrate-induced lipemia. It is a fact that experiments have been done in which subjects were fed high levels of carbohydrates, and it is a fact that in some of these experiments [33,84] the subjects' blood fat levels have increased. The tricky point (and the one many observers have missed) is that the carbohydrate fed to these people was sucrose—simple sugar. Similar experiments done with sugarless bread (which is a starchy carbohydrate containing, among other ingredients, ground wheat) showed that not only did the fats *not* increase, they significantly decreased.[33,84] It thus turns out that while simple carbohydrates (as in cupcakes) do indeed raise blood fats, complex carbohydrates (as in lima beans) do not. They make them go down.

Therefore carbohydrate-induced lipemia is only a concern in the case of simple carbohydrates. If you hear someone say that carbohydrates cause blood fats to increase, it can be deduced that he is correct only insofar as he is talking about simple carbohydrates, not complex carbohydrates.

There is another point that we mentioned in discussing diabetes and that we should emphasize once again here. This has to do with the difference in how the body handles starches as opposed to simple sugars. When you eat starches, the first thing your digestive tract does is to break the complex starch down into the simple sugars of which it is composed. In getting the energy out of these starches, your body cells need first to have them broken down into simple sugars, because only these simple sugars can be used directly by the cell for energy. So you might very reasonably ask: What is the difference? If the body is going to break them down into simple sugars anyway, why not save it all the trouble and eat simple sugars in the first place? That is a good question, and the answer has several parts. First, simple sugars are devoid of vitamins and other essential nutrients, whereas the complex starches that you eat, such as lima beans, bread, and so forth, will not only be composed of sugars for energy but will also have the many needed nutrients. Second, experience tells us that simple sugars will raise your blood fats and make you put on weight, whereas the complex starches will not. Third, when you eat simple sugars, the sugar gets into your bloodstream at a very high rate—so fast, in fact, that your pancreas, in effect, overreacts, producing *more* insulin than is really needed to metabolize the consumed sugar. The result is that your blood sugar will often be driven to lower than normal levels before the pancreas can be turned off once again, and you may find yourself experiencing the uncomfortable signs of hypoglycemia: weakness, depression, and perhaps dizziness.

So it is pretty clear that when someone tells you that it is silly to avoid sugar because the body cannot live without sugar, he's off on the wrong track. The body definitely needs sugar, it is true, but it needs sugar at complex starch rates, not at candy bar rates.

Amino Acids (Proteins)

Geophysicists tell us that billions of years ago there was no life on our planet, only raging seas and a gaseous atmosphere full of chemicals. These seas were there and the chemicals were there as an evolutionary result of the earth cooling off from a mass of hot gas to a mass of rock, water, and chemicals. Among these chemicals were some called amino acids, simple compounds made up of nitrogen, carbon, oxygen, hydrogen, and sometimes sulphur. Some people believe that these acids in the right environment were responsible for spontaneously organizing, as a result of random motion, into the first forms of life in this world; that from these first life-forms all the life-forms that today exist on the earth were slowly evolved.

Amino acids can be found in every form of life on the planet, animal or plant. In living things amino acids play many important roles, but no doubt the most important role is as a building block for proteins. All proteins are made up of long—incredibly long—strings of amino acids of several different kinds. And there are literally billions and trillions of different kinds of proteins. Although there are only about 20 amino acids that can go into making up proteins, there are unaccountably many varieties of proteins that can be constructed from these few amino acid building blocks: by making long chains of them, short chains, varying the order of the amino acids in the chain, and so on.

If amino acids are the basic building blocks of living cells, then you would have to call proteins the rooms, walls, vehicles, equipment, and fixtures of living cells constructed from these building blocks. Protein is everywhere: in our muscles, bones, eyes, hair—everywhere. In fact, 60 percent of the dry weight of a human being is protein.

Since the proteins in our body are different from those in any other living species, it is clear that our body must have some way to manufacture them. And this is the case. Our cells manufacture needed proteins from simple amino acid building blocks. However, the amino acids themselves cannot be manufactured. They must be eaten as part of the diet. Basically our bodies will take any protein that is eaten—from whatever source (plants or animals) and no matter how complex—and will break it down in the digestive tract into its component amino acids. When this is done the amino acids are passed along to the various cells which then assemble them into whatever types of protein the cells need.

Although our body cells are incapable of manufacturing any amino acids from scratch there is a considerable capability in the cells to manufacture some amino acids from others. And, in fact, out of all the amino acids that can be found in human protein, there are only eight that cannot be manufactured from any other amino acids. However, these eight can themselves be converted into any one of the remaining amino acids. These eight amino acids are called essential amino acids, because our body cells can be healthy *only* if they have access to all eight of them. The eight essential amino acids are:

Leucine	Methionine
Isoleucine	Phenylalanine
Valine	Threonine
Lysine	Tryptophane

These eight amino acids are the only amino acids that you need to know about. From the point of view of bodily needs, there are no others.

In order for a cell to build a particular protein molecule, all of the essential amino acids that go into making up that protein have to be available at the same time. If some of these amino acids were not in the food that was eaten, then the protein cannot be built. Furthermore, the job cannot wait until the next day in hopes that a new meal will bring the missing amino acids. By the next day the previous day's amino acids have either been used for protein or energy or have been excreted. They are not saved. It is thus vital that meals in general be complete in terms of amino acids eaten. That is, it is vital, in general, that a meal have all eight of the essential amino acids, not just some of them. Now, of course, it does not hurt to have an incomplete meal now and then or even to skip a meal altogether from time to time. But what does hurt is to have incomplete meals as a matter of habit.

To a certain extent it is not very practical to think in terms of the amino acids you eat. After all, most of us think about food when we eat. We think about beef or beans or bread or milk, but we do not think about amino acids. So the important thing to know is whether or not the food we eat or intend to eat has all the essential amino acids we need and in needed quantities. If it does not, we had better make a change. If it does, well and good; we are on the right track.

As you might suppose, anyone eating a broad variety of grains, vegetables, and meats cannot help getting all the essential amino acids. There is no way around it. And in fact, a survey of the essential amino acid contents of unprocessed foods reveals that it is really very hard to find a diet that is both sufficient in calories and deficient in the essential amino acids.[110,111,112] In other words, no matter how peculiar or narrow a diet may be, as long as it consists of unprocessed foods and provides enough calories to sustain life, it is not likely to be deficient in amino acids. This is contrary to the popular belief that some foods are incomplete in terms of amino acids while others are complete.

Many people have the idea that protein is the answer to everything. If people are starving in Africa, the most common response is to send them a shipment of protein. As we have already pointed out, protein is needed everywhere in the body—it is certainly a good thing. But it is possible to get too much of a good thing. What the body needs most each day is energy to keep the cell factories running. Protein (that is, amino acids), vitamins, and other elements are needed in smaller amounts for the factories' growth, "lubrication," and so forth. But when protein is eaten in excess of the amount needed for cell growth and repair, the body must work hard to convert this excess protein to a form that can be used for energy. Not only does the body have to perform extra work to get the protein converted over to fuel, which in itself might not be so bad, but there is also the problem of cholesterol and fats that are usually present in a high-protein diet. From Chapter 3 we know where *that* road takes us: heart disease, diabetes, and other degenerative diseases.

The point is, you do not need a lot of protein to obtain your needed amino acids. You can, for example, get all the essential amino acids necessary for healthy life by a diet composed exclusively of grains, vegetables, and fruits. The human body is an ingenious mechanism that has evolved over millions of years to derive all of its nutrients in an efficient way from the things that primitive man could lay his hands on. These things were roots, leafy things, grains, fruit, and occasionally an animal. In modern terminology this might translate to: potatoes and the like, lettuce and the like, wheat and the like, apples and the like, and an occasional baked halibut. But two pounds of steak each day is clearly not a diet for which our bodies evolved.

Vitamins *

During the cold December of 1911, a young Polish biochemist named Casimir Funk was deeply absorbed in his study of several great and puzzling health problems. Four destructive diseases were then widespread in the world: beriberi, pellagra, rickets, and scurvy. Funk spent his time poring over the literature about these diseases, studying where they occurred, under what conditions they could be

* A large portion of the information in this section was abstracted from the classic work by Wagner and Folkers on vitamins and coenzymes. (See reference 115.)

cured, who had them and who did not. The more he studied, the more firmly Funk came to believe that the causes of these diseases could be nothing else than something wrong with the nutrition of the people who contracted them. He could have concluded that people with these diseases were somehow getting poisons in the food they were eating or that they were victims of a viral contagion. But the data simply would not support these conclusions. Funk was forced to conclude that these diseases—all four of them— were caused by something vital that was missing from the foods people ate. Furthermore, his data showed him that the missing ingredient, whatever it was, had to be different for each of the four diseases.

It was thus that Casimir Funk, in a flurry of creative reasoning, composed his now famous theory of vitamins. Funk proposed that four vital elements, which he named vitamins, were contained in astonishingly minute quantities in nutritious foods. If any one of these vitamins were left out of a person's food, the person would contract the disease associated with that vitamin. Funk was 100 percent correct in his conclusion, even though he had no idea whatever what these vitamins might be. But he knew they must exist. It was not until years later that the vitamins were finally isolated and chemically identified. Today we know the chemical structure of all four of the vitamins, as well as a lot about how they work. Scurvy is caused by a vitamin C deficiency; pellagra is caused by a niacinamide deficiency; beriberi is caused by a vitamin B deficiency; and rickets is caused by a vitamin D deficiency. Vitamins B, C, and D, and niacinamide are essential ingredients for good nutrition, even though they are needed only in extremely small amounts.

We have been talking about vitamins for only two paragraphs, and already some confusion has been generated. Why, you might ask, were three of the vitamins associated with three of the above diseases given alphabetical letter names, while the fourth was given some chemical name? Furthermore, what happened to the letter A? These are good questions. To start with, Funk himself did not assign letters to his vitamins at all. He named vitamins after the disease they cured. For example, he called vitamin B the antiberiberi vitamin, not vitamin B. The letter designations came later on when the vitamins were assigned letters on the basis of some of their chemical properties. This might have been all right if things had proceeded more slowly in vitamin chemistry but it did not work out that way.

During the 1930s and 1940s it was found that a great many chemicals in minute quantities are needed in our food to keep us healthy. As these chemicals were discovered they were given letter names, not on a sequential basis but on the basis of some aspect of the chemical's properties. For instance, the letter K was given to a coagulation-promoting chemical because K was the first letter in the Scandinavian word *koagulation*. Other letter assignments were made on the basis of similar inconsequential considerations. Soon everything got mixed up. Vitamins were named out of order; some got letters, some chemical names, and confusion prevailed.

The B vitamins are particularly confusing. If you look ahead at Table II, you will find four kinds of vitamin B, namely: B_1, B_2, B_6, and B_{12}, each with its own chemical name in addition to its letter designation.

These are all different vitamins, and the fact that they all use the letter B is strictly an accident of history. It was originally thought that there were compelling reasons to group all these vitamins together. This is no longer the case. If we were naming them today, we would give them all separate chemical names and forget the letters and numbers altogether. Notice that B_3, B_5, B_7, B_8, B_9, B_{10}, and B_{11} are missing from the table. Except for B_9, these letters were used to name other chemicals that people originally thought were vitamins. Some of them are, in fact, still considered to be vitamins, but of lesser importance, while others have since been shown not to be vitamins. The case of B_9 is rather strange. For some reason, the designation B_9 was skipped altogether and never assigned to any chemical. Believe it or not, there are other B chemicals besides B_1 through B_{12}. They also have either been shown to be unimportant, or else their activity as a human vitamin is still somewhat questionable. These others are B_{12a}, B_{12b}, B_{12c}, B_{12d}, B_{14}, B_{15}, B_c, B_p, B_t, and B_x.

The set of vitamins having a B name have been called B vitamins or the B complex vitamins. Nowadays the whole B terminology is gradually being dropped, and their regular chemical names are being used.

After a period of time, all the letters in the alphabet had been used up naming vitamins. That in itself is surprising to most people. The average person does not realize that there are so many different vitamins. At last count (and depending on whom you talk to), there were 41 kinds of vitamins. Some of this list of 41 might actually be put into the questionable category, since their importance in the human body has been difficult to determine. Among those that are known to be important, some are so common among foods that many experts tend to ignore them. They feel that a deficiency in such a vitamin would be very hard to generate and thus not worth worrying about as a vitamin. But even with these exceptions, there are still a lot of vitamins.

Which brings up a point. In the days just before Casimir Funk, it was thought that the only important ingredients of food were fat, carbohydrate, and protein. Today that seems ridiculous. It even seemed wrong to Funk. After Funk's time it might be thought that the only important ingredients in food were fat, carbohydrate, protein, and Funk's four vitamins. Today we know that this is not true. Many other vitamins and minerals (than these) are needed to support life. The question is then: Are we done today? Have we discovered all the vitamins there are to discover? The answer is undoubtedly no. There are unquestionably things in food that are vital to health but not as yet identified.

We have talked about vitamins, but we have not really said precisely what vitamins are. So here is a definition of what a vitamin is that you can hang onto. You may find it very helpful when talking to someone who knows bits of information about nutrition but does not have the whole picture. A vitamin is a chemical for which all of the following are true:

1. It is an organic chemical, rather than an inorganic chemical such as a mineral.
2. It is present in food in extremely small amounts.
3. It is essential for normal health.
4. A specific disease occurs if it is absent.
5. It cannot be made by the body.

That is a vitamin. A hormone is just like a vitamin, except that the body can make it by itself.

Most of us think of human body chemistry as being very different from that of a snail or a gopher, for example. And in many ways it is, particularly in the proteins that make up the body tissue. But interestingly enough, at the level of the vitamins, hormones, and amino acids, all forms of life are remarkably similar. Every vitamin, hormone, and amino acid in man occurs in nearly every form of life on earth, and vice versa. This is one of the strange and powerful unities of nature—that the one-celled microorganism behaves so much like the brain cell of a human. It is also interesting to note that a vitamin for one species can be a hormone for other species. For instance, ascorbic acid (vitamin C) is a vitamin for humans, because it cannot be manufactured by the cells in the human body. But it is a hormone for nearly every other form of life on the planet (except monkeys and apes), since they can all fabricate it within their own cells.

There is still a lot of uncertainty about how some vitamins work. But the primary role of many vitamins is now known. Many vitamins are used by the body as part of one of the body's many enzymes. An enzyme is a complicated chemical which acts as a specialized fabrication tool inside the cell. It may have only one job to do: to join molecules of a certain kind together. Joining two molecules together may be only one step in a long process in which some very complicated chemical is being built. But the enzyme is just like the man in the car factory that puts the front right wheel on the new cars as the assembly line moves along in front of him. All he sees are front right wheels, over and over again. He never sees an engine or an axle, just the front wheel of car after car. The enzyme is in the same boat. It does the same job over and over again for different molecules but is not really concerned with the thing that is being built.

The enzyme itself is a large protein molecule, coupled to one or two smaller molecules called coenzymes. Many vitamins are the coenzymes of various of the body's enzymes. Since the enzyme cannot work without its coenzyme, then the molecule that is being built by the enzyme cannot be finished unless that vitamin (coenzyme) is present in the body. When the vitamin is absent, the body's cell machinery begins to fail, and one of the vitamin-deficiency diseases appears.

It appears that not all vitamins are coenzymes and not all

coenzymes are vitamins, but this is probably the most important role of vitamins in the body. Actually, a vitamin does not have to be the exact coenzyme needed by the enzyme for the enzyme to use it. In fact, the chemical that has been identified in the lab as the vitamin needed for health often turns out to be just a close relative of the needed coenzyme. The body simply takes the vitamin as is, converts it to the needed coenzyme, and proceeds to go about its business. Indeed the body's machinery is pretty adaptable, and often there are a lot of substitutes that will work equally well as some certain vitamins. In the case of vitamin A, any of the chemicals—retinol, retinal, and retinoic acid—can be converted by the body cells to the needed chemicals to get vitamin A activity. That is why on the labels of different brands of vitamin pills, you may see each brand calling vitamin A by a different chemical name. If you should take the brand X vitamin pill, you might get retinol; in the brand Y vitamin pill, you might get retinoic acid. But your body can use either one to generate vitamin A activity.

Vitamin Deficiency Symptoms

The best-known and most striking of the deficiency diseases are beriberi, rickets, scurvy, pellagra—the four identified by Casimir Funk—and a fifth disease caused by vitamin A deficiency, night blindness. These five are certainly the most dramatic of the deficiency diseases. They are terribly unpleasant, and in their worst stages horrible to the extreme. But there is a lot more to vitamin deficiency than these five diseases. It is not our goal to delve into the details of all the possible symptoms of vitamin deficiency, but let us touch on some of them to make a point. The point we wish to make is this: To sustain good health your cells must have the chemicals they need to perform the jobs of tissue repair and growth in your body. If any single chemical cannot be made available, your body will bear the brunt of the lack. In the case of a lack of vitamin A, the result could be night blindness or total blindness. But even for mild deficiencies of many of the other vitamins, in combination, you can expect such things as increased susceptibility to infection, increased susceptibility to injury, mental slowness, depression, congenital malformation of babies, and many other conditions. The point is that to feel better and to be healthier and happier, total vitamin sufficiency is very necessary.

To extract nutrients from what we eat, food is pushed along the digestive tract at optimal rates of speed, and slowly the food is broken down and the nutrients are taken out. Diarrhea and constipation result when this digestive conveyor belt is speeded up or slowed down. The first thing many people think to do when their conveyor speed is out of kilter is to take some medicine to solve the problem. In the case of constipation, for example, they might take a laxative, a harsh chemical that irritates the intestinal cells and gets the intestinal conveyor belt speeded up again. This ignores the problem of why the intestinal cells are behaving as they are. A great deal of evidence has been accumulated that shows that many intestinal problems of this kind are caused simply by faulty nutrition. The vitamin pantothenic acid is known to bring back proper elimination in many cases.[113]

Roger Williams, a noted biochemist (and in fact the discoverer of vitamin B_3), has gathered data for years on the subject of alcoholism and nutrition. There is evidence to show that the initiation and maintenance of alcoholism may be due primarily to inadequate nutrition. It is interesting to note that in studies with mice that are given free access to alcohol, those given a diet mildly deficient in certain vitamins consume more alcohol than those on a nutritionally adequate diet.

In line with the work done on alcohol, it has been found that the amount of sugar that people eat is also a function of vitamin inadequacy. In experiments done with children, it was found that children on a properly designed diet, eat, by choice, less candy than those on a vitamin-deficient diet. This experiment has been duplicated with mice as well.

Williams refers to this as "body wisdom." What he means by this is that our bodies have a natural bent to crave the things that are good for it and to reject those things that are not.[113] This is our natural body wisdom. It is clear, however, that body wisdom can be dimmed appreciably by malnutrition. Wise decisions on what to eat are easiest when the body is in the best health and hardest when the body's health is worst. The child who is malnourished—the one who most needs proper nutrients—will thus select candy to eat, while the child who is properly nourished and who can actually do without nutrients better than the malnourished child, may by choice eat something other than candy.

Clearly body wisdom is a thing to encourage. It promotes upward spirals to health, whereas its lack is the hallmark of the downward spiral to ill health.

Important Vitamins

There is no reason in the world why you should have any vitamin deficiencies, provided your diet consists principally of unrefined foods.* We use the word refined to mean any process that changes food's chemical content. Clearly some refinement changes can be small and of no consequence, while other refinement changes can completely obliterate all the nutrients in a product other than the calories. If you eat no refined foods, you will surely have no nutrient de-

* One exception is a vegetarian who eats no animal or dairy products. Some vitamin B_{12} would be necessary as a supplement.

ficiencies. If you eat only refined foods you surely will have nutrient deficiencies. If you eat a mixture of refined and unrefined foods, your likelihood of having nutrition deficiency falls somewhere between.

It is likely that you are best off if you stay in the world of unrefined foods for the present. Perhaps in the future, when mankind knows more about the human body, things will be different. It is indeed a pity that while it should be easier to eat unrefined foods than refined foods, in today's modern society it is just the other way around.

At any rate, if you are heavily into refined foods right now, you may have a brief need for a vitamin supplement while you are getting your 2100 Program going. After three or four weeks, however, you should no longer be taking vitamin supplements. By then your body wisdom should be in full swing again, and you should be getting all of your vitamins from unrefined foods on your 2100 Program.

Table II is a list of the vitamins you might need if you are going to supplement your diet for a short time. The dosages suggested in the table are those recommended * by the National Academy of Sciences.[114] A simple, abbreviated version of Table II is shown in Table III. This abbreviated table will help you to gain a quick acquaintance with the vitamins of importance.

In using a vitamin supplement, even for a short while as should be your goal, be sure to use the dosage recommendations shown. Read the label before you purchase a supply of vitamins. If you cannot find the right combination of dosages in one brand, it is all right to buy more than one brand and take multiple doses, but be careful about overdoses. Overdosage of vitamins can be toxic, especially with

---

* The authors are not in complete agreement with the vitamin and mineral dosages of the National Academy of Sciences, whose recommended dosages in some cases appear too high.

Table II. VITAMINS AND RECOMMENDED DAILY

Note: These figures cover people of average size and weight at each age.

	Age (Years)	Vit. A. (Units)	Vit. D (Units)	Vit. E (Units)	Vit. C (mg)
Infants	0–⅙	1500	400	5	35
	⅙–½	1500	400	5	35
	½–1	1500	400	5	35
Children	1–2	2000	400	10	40
	2–3	2000	400	10	40
	3–4	2500	400	10	40
	4–6	2500	400	10	40
	6–8	3500	400	15	40
	8–10	3500	400	15	40
Males	10–12	4500	400	20	40
	12–14	5000	400	20	45
	14–18	5000	400	25	55
	18–22	5000	400	30	60
	22–35	5000	—	30	60
	35–55	5000	—	30	60
	55–75+	5000	—	30	60
Females	10–12	4500	400	20	40
	12–14	5000	400	20	45
	14–16	5000	400	25	50
	16–18	5000	400	25	50
	18–22	5000	400	25	55
	22–35	5000	—	25	55
	35–55	5000	—	25	55
	55–75+	5000	—	25	55
Pregnancy		6000	400	30	60
Lactation		8000	400	30	60
Result of Deficiency (Selected):		Night Blindness	Rickets	Red Blood Cell Rupture	Scurvy

* See Table III for a definition of dosage measures.

DOSAGES*
Exceptions can be scaled up or down accordingly.

Folacin (mg)	Niacin (mg-equivalents)	Riboflavin (Vit. B_2) (mg)	Thiamin (Vit. B_1) (mg)	Pyridoxin (Vit. B_6) (mg)	Cobalamin (Vit. B_{12}) (mcg)
.05	5	.4	.2	.2	1.0
.05	7	.5	.4	.3	1.5
.1	5	.6	.5	.4	2.0
.1	8	.6	.6	.5	2.0
.2	8	.7	.6	.6	2.5
.2	9	.8	.7	.7	3.0
.2	11	.9	.8	.9	4.0
.2	13	1.1	1.0	1.0	4.0
.3	15	1.2	1.1	1.2	5.0
.4	17	1.3	1.3	1.4	5.0
.4	18	1.4	1.4	1.6	5.0
.4	20	1.5	1.5	1.8	5.0
.4	18	1.6	1.4	2.0	5.0
.4	18	1.7	1.4	2.0	5.0
.4	17	1.7	1.3	2.0	5.0
.4	14	1.7	1.2	2.0	6.0
.4	15	1.3	1.1	1.4	5.0
.4	15	1.4	1.2	1.6	5.0
.4	16	1.4	1.2	1.8	5.0
.4	15	1.5	1.2	2.0	5.0
.4	13	1.5	1.0	2.0	5.0
.4	13	1.5	1.0	2.0	5.0
.4	13	1.5	1.0	2.0	5.0
.4	13	1.5	1.0	2.0	6.0
.8	15	1.8	+.1	2.5	8.0
.5	20	2.0	+.5	2.5	6.0
Anemia	Pellagra	Growth Retardation	Beriberi	Skin Disease	Pernicious Anemia

A and D. If you are of average size and weight for your age, the dosages in Table II are considered safe. If you are not of average size and weight for your age, dosages need to be scaled accordingly.

Table III. VITAMINS AND RECOMMENDED DOSAGES* (ABBREVIATED)

Vitamin	Daily Dosage *	Results of Deficiency (Selected)
A	5000 units	Night Blindness
D	400 units	Rickets
E	30 units	Red Blood Cell Rupture
C	60-mg	Scurvy
Folacin	.4 mg	Anemia
Niacin	15 mg-equivalents	Pellagra
Riboflavin (B_2)	1.6 mg	Growth Retardation
Thiamin (B_1)	1.3 mg	Beriberi
Pyridoxin (B_6)	2 mg	Skin Disease
Cobalamin (B_{12})	5 mcg	Pernicious Anemia

* Dosages are measured in units, in milligrams (mg's), and in micrograms (mcg's). Each of these measures are fractions of an ounce. In particular:

1 unit = 3/280,000,000 ounce
1 mg = 1/28,000 ounce
1 mcg = 1/28,000,000 ounce

Ordinarily one does not have to know what these measures are in order to buy vitamin tablets. Most manufacturers state the vitamin dosage using exactly the same measures we have shown, so all one must do is purchase a brand or combination of brands that give approximately the numbers desired.

Essential Minerals

Like vitamins, essential minerals are chemicals that the body's cells need to perform well. In fact, many minerals act as coenzymes just as vitamins do. But unlike vitamins, which are fairly complex chemicals, the essential minerals are very simple chemicals. In addition, minerals are all inorganic substances such as can be dug out of rock, while vitamins are organic substances found in living things. Other than these two differences, however, the essential minerals are like vitamins. They are vital to the health of every body cell, and if one of them is absent from the diet, specific deficiency symptoms appear.

Table IV lists all the minerals that are considered to be essential and the dosages recommended by the National Academy of Sciences.[114] Actually, there are a lot more minerals necessary to good health than those we have shown in this short list, but the others are so plentiful in our food supply (compared to the amounts needed), that it is very unlikely that anyone would ever become deficient in any of them. Since Table IV is a fairly complicated table, we have included a very simple abbreviation of it, Table V, that will give you the general idea of minerals and dosages.

Of course if you are eating a broad selection of fruits, vegetables, and so on, it is extremely improbable that you would be deficient in any of the essential minerals. If this is the case, keep up the good work; you are on the right track. You are no doubt already feeling happy, alert, and strong. But if your diet contains a high proportion of highly processed foods, then a mineral supplement could probably do you some good. Like a vitamin supplement, a mineral supplement will help you to develop your body wisdom, your natural tendency to eat the sort of things that are good for you and to reject the things that are not so good. The real objective in the long run is to get you eating the deli-

Table IV. ESSENTIAL MINERALS AND RECOMMENDED DOSAGES

NOTE: These figures cover people of average size and weight at each age. Exceptions can be scaled up or down accordingly.

	Age (Years)	Calcium (mg)	Phosphorus (mg)	Magnesium (mg)	Iodine (mcg)	Iron (mg)
Infants	0–⅙	400	200	40	25	6
	⅙–½	500	400	60	40	10
	½–1	600	500	70	45	15
Children	1–2	700	700	100	55	15
	2–3	800	800	150	60	15
	3–4	800	800	200	70	10
	4–6	800	800	200	80	10
	6–8	900	900	250	100	10
	8–10	1000	1000	250	110	10
Males	10–12	1200	1200	300	125	10
	12–14	1400	1400	350	135	18
	14–18	1400	1400	400	150	18
	18–22	1800	1800	400	140	10
	22–35	1800	1800	350	140	10
	35–55	1800	1800	350	125	10
	55–75+	1800	1800	350	110	10
Females	10–12	1200	1200	300	110	18
	12–14	1300	1300	350	115	18
	14–16	1300	1300	350	120	18
	16–18	1300	1300	350	115	18
	18–22	1800	1800	350	100	18
	22–35	1800	1800	300	100	18
	35–55	1800	1800	300	90	18
	55–75+	1800	1800	300	80	10
Pregnancy		+400	+400	450	125	18
Lactation		+500	+500	450	150	18
Symptoms of Deficiency (Selected)		Bone Disease	Muscular Convulsions	Growth Retardation	Goiter	Anemia

Table V. ESSENTIAL MINERALS AND
RECOMMENDED DOSAGES
(ABBREVIATED)

Mineral	Dosage	Symptoms of Deficiency (Selected)
Calcium	800 mg	Bone Disease
Phosphorus	800 mg	Muscular Convulsions
Magnesium	325 mg	Growth Retardation
Iodine	120 mg	Goiter
Iron	14 mg	Anemia

cious assortment of things that nature has to offer. A mineral supplement will help your body wisdom grow so that this objective of eating all of nature's bounties will tend to happen more easily and naturally. But in the same way that a vitamin supplement is to be viewed only as a short-term affair, a mineral supplement is also to be viewed as temporary (a matter of weeks), while your new eating habits are being established.

In selecting a brand of mineral tablets, take time to read the ingredients label carefully to be certain that you are getting all of the minerals shown. Since minerals are very cheap compared to vitamins, you usually do not have to worry about being short-changed by the manufacturer, as far as amount is concerned. It is all right to buy more than one brand, if necessary, to get the recommended quantities, but be careful of overdosages.

Essential Fatty Acids

We have spent a lot of time in this book discussing the bad things that happen if you eat too much fat. When you consider that the average American eats the equivalent in fat of more than a cup of shortening each day, it is certainly no wonder that fat is a problem. But it turns out that some fat is absolutely necessary for good health. However, the amount of fat needed is laughably small. You need only a few drops of fat per day to get all you need. You can easily satisfy your body's need for fat by eating fruit, vegetables, and/or grain. A few spoonfuls of oatmeal, for example, supply all the fat you need for a day.[116]

Although the body needs fats in order to use its fat-soluble vitamins A, D, and E, the fat it needs for these purposes can be manufactured internally.[115] Fats do not have to be eaten for this purpose.

In 1932, it was found, however, that even with plenty of fats for the fat-soluble vitamins, a kind of fat deficiency disease could develop in mice.[115] Later it was found that similar disease conditions would also occur in human beings. But if certain vegetable fats were added to the diet in minute amounts, the disease disappeared. The vegetable fats found to eliminate the disease are called *essential* fats. Six essential fats were discovered. All six are not needed for health, however, just one. The kind of fat that was found to be most effective among these six is that which is formed from linoleic acid.

You need not concern yourself with taking essential fat supplements or essential fatty acid supplements. You do not need them, unless you eat absolutely nothing in the way of fruit or vegetables or grains, and on the 2100 Program this is not possible.

Unidentified Essential Chemicals

On page 89, a pie chart was drawn which showed all the chemicals necessary for nutrition broken up into six classes. One of these six classes was labeled "Unidentified Essential Chemicals." What are these unidentified chemicals, and how many are there? Since they are still unidentified, we of

The Role of Nutrients

course have no way of knowing. But you can be sure that there are plenty of chemicals that are still in this class. We have not discovered all the vitamins, that is undoubtedly true. Therefore, this sixth class must contain some unidentified vitamins. It may also contain minerals or essential fats. We will simply have to wait to see what else science discovers.

As time passes the chemicals that are in this "unidentified" class will gradually be identified; when they are, they will move out of this class of unknowns into one of the other classes. In the meantime, the existence of this class is a good lesson for all of us. The lesson is this: Until science learns all there is to know about the human body, it does not behoove us to take chances on the food we eat. It is unwise, for example, to live on food that has had the good refined out of it and then "enriched" with chemicals. No matter what is put back into the food as enrichment, we can be fairly sure that all of the chemicals in the sixth class, by definition, will be missing. Rather, the wiser course is to eat a broad variety of natural, unrefined foodstuffs. We then can be certain that we will be consuming what we need, because this is the sort of thing upon which the human race has grown up. The chemicals that our bodies need—both the known chemicals and the unidentified ones—are more likely to be in this wide variety of natural foodstuffs than anywhere else we could look.

CHAPTER 5

Other Players in the Game of Health

In the last four chapters we did a lot of work building up our knowledge of the cause and prevention of degenerative diseases. We also worked hard learning about vitamins, amino acids, and other chemicals needed for good health. In this chapter we are going to be able to put some of this knowledge to use. There are many groups which directly affect your health: the food industry, the medical profession, the health food people, and the fad diet people, to mention a few. Are they helping you or hurting you?

The Food Industry: Unhealthy for Children and Other Living Things

The next few paragraphs may be distasteful to some readers. To emphasize an important point about the quality of food that is available to you on your grocer's shelves, we are going to speak about food and about garbage all in the same breath. If your sensitivities are overly offended while reading this section, please feel free to skip over to the next section, with the simple admonition in mind that what you think is good for you at your supermarket may not be so good after all, and some care may have to be exercised in finding beneficial foods on your supermarket's shelves.

When you buy a potato at your supermarket, you are buying food, food that can nourish your body. But if the potato is left around long enough it will spoil, and then it will no longer nourish your body: it may even become poisonous. Then it is no longer food. It has become garbage and is fit only for your disposal. When food has been changed so that it no longer nourishes your body or becomes dangerous to your health, we call it garbage. That is how garbage is defined.

Using this definition (that garbage is simply food that has been changed to render it harmful), let us see what we can learn about supermarket products. You will probably be surprised to discover that, by our definition, much of what is being sold as food on your supermarket's shelves is not really food at all. It is garbage. It is garbage handsomely packaged and labeled as food, but it is garbage all the same.

Bread is a food staple made from flour, which has been a source of nutrients for man as long as there has been a written history. But go to the bread section of your supermarket and take a look at what has been done to this time-honored food. You will find row upon row of sugary, bleached breads that are so devoid of nutrients that even cereal weevils cannot maintain life on them. Such breads are no longer capable of maintaining human life,* and given the large amounts of sugar that many of them contain, they are worse than simply neutral: They are actually harmful to health

---

* There was a time when a man could be sentenced to a long jail term on bread and water and could live to tell about it. But today, with many of our modern breads, a long jail term on bread and water would be equivalent to a death sentence.

LIVE LONGER NOW 118

(as we learned in the discussion of the role that sugar plays in raising blood fats and causing diabetes). These breads are therefore not food; they are garbage and should be put into the disposal.

It is sad but true that through the use of highly emotional television commercials, food manufacturers have become wizards at making garbage seem attractive and even exciting to eat. If you walk over to the soft drink section of the supermarket you will recognize soft drinks that you have seen advertised on television in stirringly dramatic commercial spots. In fact, you may find yourself feeling stirred up all over again just by being in the soft drink section with these "glorious" products. But what do you find if you investigate the contents of a leading soft drink? You find that the product contains carbonated sugar water, phosphoric acid, caffeine, coloring, and flavoring. Sugar has a role in causing diabetes, caffeine has a role in the cause of heart disease, and phosphoric acid is a potent chemical for dissolving tooth enamel.* So then what has this glorious product got to offer the person (often a youngster) who buys it? It has a known role in the cause of diabetes, heart disease, and tooth decay. Like the rotten potato, it is garbage that should be thrown out.

But let us not stop at soft drinks. Many other products are just as bad. Find the cookie section, for example. Remember those powerful ads on television about the boy and his cookies? The cookie people would have you believe through the power of suggestion that the cookies being advertised were essential to a boy's happiness during youth. But based on its ingredients list, these cookies are really good for cavities, diabetes, and heart disease—just like the soft drink.

---

* A tooth left in a cola drink overnight will in most cases have all of its enamel dissolved. This is an experiment you can easily duplicate at home with discarded baby teeth and your favorite cola drink.

Other Players in the Game of Health

The list of sweet things like cookies and soft drinks goes on and on. We do not have to enumerate them here. They are listed on your supermarket's shelves. Let us instead skip over to the breakfast cereals and see what we find.

The cereal corporations are responsible for manufacturing and promoting an incredible line of breakfast garbage. These corporations prey on the minds of children, who are brainwashed with fervent intensity. Surely no child who watches Saturday morning cartoons on television can help but feel he would be lots better off in life if he were eating one of the fancifully named cereals that are advertised before and after each cartoon. If you have a child between the ages of 4 and 12, ask him or her what kind of cereals would be fun to eat. You may be amazed at the string of cereals your child can rattle off.

There appear to be three major cereal manufacturers that are involved in this Saturday morning escapade with children, which we shall refer to as Corporation A, Corporation B, and Corporation C. (If you want to find out the true identities of these corporations, a visit to the cereals section of your supermarket will provide you with their names. You will recognize them as old-line, respected food companies.)

Corporation A manufactures a cereal which we shall call by the code name Sugar Yums, but which you can find under its real name at the Supermarket. Its ingredients list is: sugar; oat flour; "degermed" yellow cornmeal; corn syrup; salt; coconut and peanut oil; chemicals to produce color, taste and consistency; preservatives; and vitamins. The "good" ingredients in Sugar Yums are evidently supposed to be the oat flour and the cornmeal. But sugar has been added to these things, and in such quantity that sugar is the largest single ingredient of this cereal. Knowing what we know about sugar and its relation to diabetes and heart disease, we would have to say that whatever food was in this cereal to begin with has been changed so that it no longer is nourishing and is, in fact, harmful. Sugar Yums, like the bread and the sweets mentioned above, is therefore not food at all, but garbage. Even without the sugar, Sugar Yums would be highly suspect, since the addition of vitamins to the cereal also mentioned on the label indicates that the primary ingredients—flour and cornmeal—had had some of their nutritional chemicals refined out of them. Adding chemicals back would be all right, if we could be certain that they were all added back. But we cannot be certain. In fact, we can be certain that *not* all essential chemicals were added back. In addition, Sugar Yums has other irrelevant chemical additives for taste, color, consistency, and preservation which are possibly harmful. Therefore, even without the sugar, it is possible—even probable—that Sugar Yums has been changed from food to garbage, and with the sugar thrown in, there is no question: It is garbage.

The list of garbage products manufactured by Corporation A is a long one. But so are the lists for Corporations B and C. Corporation B manufactures a breakfast cereal that we shall call by the code name Super Wows,* in which the largest ingredient is sugar, the third largest is corn syrup, and the fourth largest is honey. In order of quantity, three of the four largest components of Super Wows are thus simple sugars. Almost as an afterthought Corporation B has placed the "cereal" part of this product, namely wheat, in the number two spot. Assuming that they began with wheat, it is clear that this company was successful at manufacturing garbage from it. The additive problem with this product is the same as it is for the Corporation A product above.

Corporation C manufactures a breakfast cereal that we

---

* If you are thinking by this time that these code names are in any way extravagant in their silliness, you owe it to yourself to check out the actual names of children's cereals. Extravagant silliness in their naming seems to be their hallmark.

shall call Sugar Drops. In this product simple sugars are far and away the largest ingredients. The wheat that is supposed to make up this cereal has obviously been converted from food to garbage—just like all the above cereals. And as a side comment, we notice the problem of additives also applies here: too many questionable chemicals put into the cereal, and too many essential chemicals taken out.

We have mentioned three particular cereal products of the corporations that apparently are the leading cereal manufacturers. And we have seen that these three products are worse than merely not nutritious—they are actually harmful. Lest you think we have found only a few particularly extreme cases among manufactured cereals, let us hasten to add that nearly all cereals manufactured by these leaders suffer from the same problems to a greater or lesser degree. That is, the large majority of cereals on the market rely heavily on sugar as an ingredient, use highly processed foodstuffs that often require vitamin enrichment, and contain a host of additives the use of which is of questionable value to health. One wonders if these companies manufacture anything *but* garbage.

The cereal companies, however, are not the only companies manufacturing garbage. Wander through your supermarket sometime and read the labels of other products. You will find fats or sugars or myriads of additives on hundreds of other products. Do not forget the people who push dairy products that are saturated with fats and cholesterol. Nor should you forget the meat people who are able to present you with steaks so marbled with fats for tenderness that nearly three-quarters of the edible portion of a T-bone steak today is fat [*] (not counting the water content of the steak). All of these individuals are in the

---

[*] See Composition of Foods in the Appendix.

business of turning out products whose effect on your body is harmful and therefore should be labeled as garbage, not food.

You can even find garbage being sold as baby food by the most respected of companies. One company, which we shall call Baby Formula, Inc., has recently begun advertising a new product to which we shall assign the code name Formula X. Formula X is intended for the use of babies who are four months old and older. From the chemical analysis and ingredients list on the label, it appears that at least 20 percent (perhaps as high as 50 percent) of the carbohydrate in Formula X is plain table sugar. Formula X is intended to be a major part of a baby's diet for some period of time. It seems inescapable that a nationwide use of this amount of sugar in babies' diets could lead to a high national incidence of early diabetes. Therefore, Formula X is not a healthy thing to eat and must be classified as garbage just like Sugar Drops, Super Wows, the rotten potato, and all the rest.

The long and short of it is that food products in your supermarket, particularly those that are being heavily promoted, tend to be harmful rather than beneficial to your health. Sugar, fats, and salt are often major parts of food products. In fact, one has to really put his mind to it to be able to find products at the supermarket that are not spoiled by these ingredients. (Is it any wonder that degenerative diseases are a problem of epidemic proportions in this country?) In addition, the problem of unrestrained use of food additives is clearly present in most products. And finally, overprocessing (however that is to be defined) is clearly a major problem.

The things that you should eat and some helpful hints for supermarket shopping to insure that what you buy is what you need are presented in Part II of this book.

Fad Diets: Be Wary

In recent years, scores of books on diets for losing weight have appeared on the market. New diets or new techniques that purport to be good for losing weight seem to crop up every day, and the public's interest in these new diets and techniques is clearly very great. Millions of Americans are overweight, and most of them are looking for something that will effectively aid them in losing their unwanted fat. The processes in the body that control our ability to permanently increase or decrease our body weight are very complex, and unfortunately both the public and most of the individuals pushing new weight-loss diets and new weight-loss techniques are ignorant of these processes. As a result, misunderstanding of the causes and prevention of overweight is widespread, while weight-loss practices that are not only ineffective but even harmful abound.

The human body contains various control mechanisms, which maintain the body in some desirable state. The body has a mechanism, for example, for controlling body temperature. It is a marvelously effective control system capable of maintaining the body's temperature at 98.6 degrees most of the time. The body also has a marvelously effective control mechanism for controlling the blood sugar level at a relatively constant value. And, what is of interest to us in this section, the body has a means for controlling body weight that is normally so effective that an adult will often maintain a body weight that changes very little for 20 years, despite large variations in the needs for food that may have occurred during such a time span.

The mechanism that controls the body's weight might be likened to the mechanism that controls the temperature in your home. In your home the temperature control mechanism (namely, the thermostat) exerts control by changing the amount of heat introduced into the house. In your body the mechanism that controls body weight * (which we shall call the appestat) does so by causing you to change the amount of food that you introduce into your stomach. The appestat mechanism is a very complex control system, and it is still only partly understood. It involves environmental factors as well as emotional factors, activity level factors, and other factors. But one thing is certain: The appestat is a very powerful mechanism—so powerful, in fact, that to keep body weight down while the appestat level is set too high is a feat of the greatest difficulty. If a person's appestat level is set too high, then he will be likely to gain weight, despite the strongest of desires to the contrary.[118] The idea that overweight, or obesity, is caused by stupidity, moral weakness, or perversity is now known to be untenable with our scientific understanding of the phenomenon. Despite all the derision that a fat person must take about his weight, he often can do as little about it as a bald man can do about his lack of hair.

We do not mean to despair of effective weight loss. It is definitely possible to lose weight and to keep it off despite the fact that the appestat setting is currently too high. But it is no trivial matter, and it often requires the greatest skill of a devoted and able physician to make it happen. Help may also be sought from one of the popular franchised weight-losing organizations (Diet Watchers, Weight Watchers, etc.). These organizations achieve commendable results insofar as they are often able to help individuals lose weight at a safe rate and to retrain their eating habits. Even with outside help, however, the failure rate is high.

As far as permanent and effective weight loss goes, the following policy/conjecture has pragmatically proved suc-

* Control appears [118] to be exerted more on basic processes of metabolism than directly on body weight, but for our purposes body weight control is an adequate interpretation of what is happening.

cessful within the Longevity Foundation: "Weight loss can occur permanently only if the appestat is readjusted to a lower level; the appestat automatically readjusts itself to a more normal level when one switches to the 2100 Diet and Exercise Program." More will be said about the 2100 Program and weight control in Part II of this book. For now we shall focus on the fad diets that exist and what they do.

The fad diets and weight-loss techniques are doomed from the beginning. Their understanding of the physiology of overweight and obesity is usually zero, and their ability to provide the way for taking weight off and keeping it off is no better. Jean Mayer, Harvard professor of nutrition, in his book *Overweight* provides us with a penetrating look at some of the fad diets and methods that have been widely touted in newspaper and magazine advertisements in recent years. We find that most advertisements are misleading, and some are simply fraudulent. Mayer quotes a postal official as saying: "Medical frauds today are more lucrative than any other criminal activity. . . . Reducing schemes are perhaps the most lucrative of such schemes."

The fad reducing diets floating around the office these days appear to fall into one of the following four categories:

1. Low-calorie diets;
2. Starvation diets;
3. Metabolism-fooling diets;
4. Low carbohydrate diets.

Low-calorie diets are the only diets used extensively by reputable weight-loss clinics. In any weight-loss clinic the most important part of the clinic's service is the creation of a low-calorie diet plan that is tailor-made for the individual who wants to lose weight. It takes into account his metabolism rate, his activity level, his need for essential chemicals, and perhaps even his food likes and dislikes. In addition, the patient's results are carefully monitored, and the diet plan is appropriately modified to account for progress or regression along the road to lower weight. With luck the individual will end up with both fewer pounds and a lower appestat level.

The problem with most of the fad reducing diets of the low-calorie type is that they are not tailored to the individual. They do not account for individual variations, and can expose an individual to a diet regimen that does not provide the basic nutrients needed for good health. An individual may get thinner, but he may also get ill. The "350 Calorie Pilot's Diet" is an example. This diet, which is touted for one and all, is only 350 calories per day, consisting of a glass of milk, an egg, three ounces of meat, and seven ounces of dressingless salad. While the diet may be adequate to maintain health for a short time for some users, it is likely to be extremely inadequate for others, particularly for those employed in heavy labor. In addition, the egg a day in this diet will adversely affect the cholesterol level.

Fasting or starvation diets are considered valuable by some people not only for losing pounds, but also as a means for resetting the appestat level. The belief is that fasting (absolutely no food) will somehow permanently alter the individual's appestat setting so that when the normal diet is resumed, the body weight will stabilize at a more normal level. Evidence available seems to indicate that fasting has undesirable effects at all levels of performance, and prolonged fasting can create physiological damage.[118] Nevertheless, the question of appestat normalization by periodic fasting is apparently still unresolved.

The "High Protein Diet" is an example of a metabolism-fooling type of diet. Promotors of the High Protein Diet believe that because protein has a higher SDA (specific dynamic action), one can eat more protein without gaining weight than carbohydrates or fat. It turns out that when a food is eaten a certain portion of that food's calories are expended just on digesting and processing it. The amount of calories expended in this way on a quantity of food is the SDA of that food. For protein the SDA is about 30 percent of the calories eaten, whereas for fat and carbohydrates, the SDAs are about 4 percent and 6 percent, respectively. This would seem to imply, for example, that 100 calories of protein would yield only about 70 calories that are accessible to be turned into fats, while for 100 calories of fat or carbohydrates, the number of calories would be 96 and 94. Trading on this phenomenon, therefore, the High Protein Diet people say that a high protein diet is really about 25 percent less capable of delivering calories into body fat than a diet containing fats and carbohydrates. But in fact, as Jean Mayer points out, when protein is mixed with carbohydrates and fat in a meal (which it almost invariably and inescapably is), then its SDA drops down to only about 5 percent rather than 30 percent.[118] That is, the body becomes much more efficient at handling protein in the presence of fat or carbohydrate, even small amounts of fat and carbohydrate. The High Protein Diet people are thus trading on a mistaken understanding of protein SDA.

Low carbohydrate diets are high in protein and especially higher in fat. If ever a diet was designed to destroy your health while reducing, this is it. High fat, of course, accelerates the development of all the degenerative diseases.

Fad reducing diets of every kind are historically and overwhelmingly unsuccessful. They are unsuccessful because they concentrate on losing weight instead of on changing the appestat level. Other techniques for losing weight such as electrical muscle stimulators, supposed "fat-dissolving enzymes," heat pads, miraculous chewing gums, and liquid potions are equally unsuccessful.

The Medical Profession

It was Benjamin Franklin who popularized that time-honored expression, "an ounce of prevention is worth a pound of cure." Any doctor will tell you that you are far better off keeping yourself healthy than recovering from an illness or accident. Your good health depends on two things: preventing yourself from getting sick in the first place, but then correcting your ills if prevention fails. Comparing prevention and correction, prevention is much more important to your well-being.

The prevention of disease primarily involves two different things. If we are talking about infective and parasitic diseases, it means defeating the germs, bugs, or viruses that cause the disease. This usually means using drugs or other forces to control the environment in which the germs, bugs, or viruses thrive. If on the other hand we are talking about degenerative diseases, it means insuring the individual's nutrition, eliminating the presence of toxic chemicals in food, and insuring the physical activity necessary for health. This does not involve the use of any drugs at all. Since degenerative diseases now account for some two thirds of all early deaths in this country, it is vital that proper prevention of them in all respects be provided for everyone.

Who is it that will make sure that effective prevention of degenerative diseases will be instituted for all? We might think that it would be the medical profession. But we would soon see that the medical profession cannot help a great deal for two reasons. First, it is so swamped with the urgent demands for *correcting* the ill health that exists that preventing ill health cannot be adequately attended to. Second, prevention entails an understanding of basic nutrition, and most physicians are undertrained in nutrition. As Professor Mayer, perhaps the most widely read and highly regarded person in his field, humorously put it: "Our studies at

Harvard among residents suggest that the average physician knows a little more about nutrition than the average secretary—unless the secretary has a weight problem. Then she probably knows more than the average physician." [119]

The medical profession is clearly a great friend of good health. But the profession's ability to institute effective programs for preventing degenerative diseases is lower than it should be. Many persons in the medical field recognize the need for change and are trying to do something about it. However, it seems unlikely that the medical profession will develop the tools and programs necessary for the effective prevention of degenerative diseases any time in the near future. Thus, for now, prevention is up to you, not your physician.

The Health Food Stores: Friend or Foe?

A few years ago health food stores were rare. Today they are everywhere and of every kind. To a great extent they are here today because people have gradually begun to realize that many of the products on their supermarket's shelves are not beneficial to their health and, indeed, may be harmful. Wanting something better for themselves, people have turned to the health food stores. The question is: Are the health food stores the answer to better nutrition?

The answer to this is both yes and no. It should first be recognized that there are many kinds of health food stores. Some specialize, for example, only in the sale of organically grown vegetables. Others specialize only in the sale of vitamins, minerals, and food supplements. Others specialize in baking and selling special kinds of natural breads. Some have a little bit of everything.

From our point of view, better nutrition for the vast majority of Americans can be accomplished in two simple ways:

1. The presence of all essential chemicals in the diet;
2. The absence, to any substantial degree, of fat, cholesterol, sugar—honey and molasses included—and salt from the diet.

From this viewpoint it is easy to evaluate the health food stores.

Every health food store that sells grain products such as bread, rolls, corn bread, and so forth is sensitive enough to its clientele to know better than to put sugar or lard into its products. However, most health food stores simply replace the sugar with other types of simple sugars—for example, honey or molasses. And the lard is simply replaced by other fats—for example, vegetable oils. Unfortunately, it is not common to find bread made simply from whole flours, water, and yeast, even in the health food store. It can be found there, however (it should hastily be added), whereas it is quite rare in the supermarket. Sadly, most of the health food breads have the serious drawback of containing large amounts of simple sugars and often large amounts of fats.

Many health food stores specialize in the sale of the essential chemicals: vitamins, minerals, amino acids, and special chemicals presumed to be essential, such as lecithin. Unless you feel you need supplements of the essential chemicals for some short period of time, you do not even need to visit this kind of store. However, if you do need a supplement, a health food store is not a bad place to get it. You can be fairly sure that good brands will be represented on the shelves. Furthermore, the persons working there will in all likelihood know a lot more about brand quality and nutrition in general than anyone working in your local supermarket or your local drugstore.

Some health food stores specialize in organically grown vegetables and other kinds of organic foods. The value of organically grown vegetables is being heavily debated.

Other Players in the Game of Health

Some people feel that if the plant grows, it must be good for you, even though it has been grown only with chemical fertilizers. Other people feel that until you know all the chemicals that are needed in human beings, you had better use animal fertilizer. The organic argument is that the only place people can for certain get all their essential chemicals is from plants, not the chemistry lab. But the only place these same plants can get all these chemicals is from the ground, and the ground is dependent nowadays upon fertilizers for its chemicals. Therefore, only with organic fertilizers can you guarantee yourself getting all your needed essential chemicals.

In the opinion of the authors of this book the organic argument is basically a sound one, although scientific substantiation is lacking. We would rate the organic vegetables being sold by organic food stores as A-1 foods. The other organic products have to be analyzed separately. If, for instance, a bread is made from organic whole grains but is also loaded with honey and vegetable oils, it can be undeniably harmful to your body.

In summary, it can be said that health food stores are an excellent source of temporarily needed chemical supplements and of some organic products. But just as in your supermarket, you've got to read the labels before you buy anything in the health food store to make sure you do not end up buying products that are harmful.

PART II
GUIDE TO GOOD HEALTH

In the chapters ahead we will learn a great deal about what foods to eat and what foods to avoid in the pursuit of good health and long life. We will learn, for example, that foods such as liver and steak, that have traditionally been considered good in any amounts, should be drastically reduced or eliminated. Upon learning this we are faced with a dilemma. Since we have long been taught to eat liver, for its iron, and steak for its protein, we must ask ourselves where our bodies will find enough iron or enough protein to meet their needs. The answer, of course, is that iron and protein can be obtained in abundance from many, many foods, and the limitations advised in this book do very little to alter the availability of iron, protein, or any other nutrient needed by the body. But in order to find out which alternate foods will supply these various nutritional needs, one must have a handbook that shows the nutritional composition of various foods.

Undoubtedly the best work in existence on the subject is Composition of Foods, *by B. K. Watt and A. L. Merrill. This 190-page handbook gives the vitamin, mineral, caloric, fat, protein and carbohydrate content of literally thousands of common kitchen foods in an easy-to-use format. This classic handbook can be obtained by writing the U.S. Department of Agriculture, or by sending $5.00 to Composition of Foods, P.O. Box 17873, Tucson, Arizona 85731. Every health-minded person should have a copy, if for no other reason than the pure fun of leafing through it to see what our everyday foods are made of.*

CHAPTER 6

Longer, Healthier Living

Nearly every person has the ability to live a long and healthful existence. Nature has given each of us an exquisitely designed body made up of more than a trillion body cells woven into an intricate network of organs, tissue, and bone. Our bodies are designed to hum along through life like well-oiled sewing machines, provided that we give them the proper foundation of food and activity for which they were designed.

For many years most Americans have been leading the "good life": a life of low physical activity and high intake of food of the wrong kind. This good life has taken away from their bodies the special foundation without which health cannot be maintained.

The good life in the United States has not been so good after all. It has produced degenerative diseases such as heart disease, atherosclerosis, and diabetes in full force. Degenerative diseases have been called a modern plague and indeed they are. Nearly 800,000 Americans will die of heart disease alone this year. And millions of other Americans will suffer from low quality health caused by degenerative diseases.

These conditions have come about because we have developed food habits and exercise habits that do not produce the necessary foundation for good health. It is time to discard these habits and build a new foundation, one that will make our bodies hum and make life as sweet as possible. The 2100 Program shows how to do this.

There are two parts to the 2100 Program: a program of eating and a program of exercise. The program of eating supplies all the ingredients your body cells need to stay healthy, and the program of exercise keeps your body's delivery systems working properly so that these ingredients will always be delivered on time and in the right amounts to the cells that need them. In the chapters that follow we shall talk about these two programs one at a time.

A Stronger Life

When you give your body the best in terms of food and exercise, your body grows strong, in return giving you back the best of which it is capable. And your body is capable of giving you amazing support in the things you want to do.

Many a person has come to a point in his job where he is not as productive as he used to be. His concentration is lower, his motivation has dropped, and his progress on the job may be depressingly unsatisfactory. Where did the old drive and energy go, he might ask? The answer is that it may have just dribbled away as his own good health was etched away by years of faulty eating and exercise patterns. Too many people fail to realize what a tremendous boon the strength of good health is to their jobs. The 2100 Program is potent medicine for getting you going on the job again. You can expect your concentration to improve and your ingenuity to be better than ever. And best of all, you can expect that the enjoyment and satisfaction you derive from your job will increase as well.

In the same way that the good health you get from the 2100 Program helps in the job situation, it also helps around the house. The energy and enthusiasm you need to tackle all those chores you have been meaning to do will be much easier to find after even a short time on the program. Your ability to organize your chores, get them done, and still find the time to relax will be significantly greater. Likewise, you may find that your enjoyment of the other members of the family will improve as your physical well-being improves.

Even your play time will be more rewarding. Think back on the times in your life when you enjoyed your recreation the very most, when your card playing, or golf, or tennis, or playing, or just plain partying was its most rewarding. The 2100 Program can put your body and mind so in tune that your play time will once more be as much fun as it was at its very best.

The 2100 Program has a way of widening your interests and broadening the things in life that give you pleasure. There is much good to be taken from life, and the 2100 Program helps one to find good things everywhere.

Longer Lifetime

The 2100 Program is a prescription for a longer, healthier life. The 2100 Program does not turn 30-year-olds into 10-year-olds to increase the length of lives; it simply helps to take away the force of degenerative diseases as a cause of death. The 2100 Program tends to stretch the middle years so that they cover the years between 40 and 80, rather than only the years from 40 to 60. It also tends to shorten the years of old age to those above 80 rather than all those years above 55 or 60.

Since the nation as a whole has never entered upon a program such as the 2100 Program, it is not known how much the average lifetime would be increased by the 2100 Program. An educated guess is that the average lifetime would take a jump of about 20 years if the 2100 Program were adopted nationally. But whether or not the 2100 Program is adopted as a national policy, its benefits are available to you if you adopt it as your policy.

A Happier Life

The last few pages have carried the message that the 2100 Program is a key to a healthier, longer life. For most persons there is also a strong carry-over affecting the degree of happiness in their lives as well. The 2100 Program gives strength and health to your body, enabling you to be a happier person. It is inevitable. When you start treating your body right your experiences take on a new life.

We do not mean to convey the impression that the 2100 Program solves all your life's problems. It cannot do that any more than anything else can. But it can grease the skids for you to solve them for yourself. A feeling of strength, vitality, and well-being in your daily life is certainly the right foundation upon which to put yourself no matter what your daily struggles.

How nice it is to wake up in the morning feeling strong and fresh, as you did as a child. How nice it is to lie down at night and fall asleep with the ease of a healthy animal. And how nice it is to be able to taste the goodness in simple foods and smell the air, the leaves, the grass in the world around you. When was the last time your body and your senses were so clear and sharp that all these sensations were part of your everyday life? For many of us it has been a long, long time. But with the 2100 Program, they can all be brought home again to us.

Life Is Today—Do It Now

With all the responsibilities that push down on us in our daily lives, there is not room for everything we want to do. We have to pick and choose what we will include in our days. It is easy for us to put off something that we would like to do or that is good for us. We can put it off again and again until somehow too much of life has slipped by, and it becomes too late to do it at all. With so much to do every day, we can easily put off actually living and experiencing our lives until some time in the future.

The 2100 Program is a way to put living back into your life. It is a way to bring life's pleasures to you now, not at some future date when you may not be here or when you may be too ill to enjoy it.

The 2100 Program takes some of your time and some of your attention. But it gives back to you richer, healthier living: a good exchange. Now is the time to start the 2100 Program. Not next year when your bills are paid off or next month when you move to your new house, but now. Wherever you are or whatever you are doing, the time to start is now.

CHAPTER 7

The 2100 Food Program

> Historically, the science of nutrition developed with a concern for hunger. And the nutrition science had only one aspect: malnutrition. Well, something snuck up on us in the U.S. and in other rich countries in the 20th century . . . the affluent society. And this presented an entirely different kind of malnutrition. Eating too much and eating the wrong kinds of food.
>
> JEREMIAH STAMLER, M.D.,
> *Chicago Health Research Foundation*

> We were born, really, to be field animals. To rise with the sun . . . to eat only when hunger dictates.
> PAUL DUDLEY WHITE, M.D.,
> *Harvard Medical School*

THE PROBLEM

Before 1900 the average American had comparatively little to choose from in his daily diet. He or his neighbors grew much of what he ate, and he got a few staples from the general store. Today the average American can choose from among more than 10,000 slickly packaged products in his supermarket. Today nearly half of his calories come from fat, and about half of the rest come from simple sugars.

Today Americans are experiencing an outbreak of degenerative diseases of epidemic proportions. Since 1900 deaths due to heart attacks have increased 500 percent, those due to diabetes have increased 250 percent. While degenerative disease death rates are out of control here, in many societies they are very low. Degenerative disease death rates are low in Japan, Italy, and Greece, and they are nearly zero in most primitive societies.

Malnutrition means bad nutrition, and bad nutrition can happen in the midst of plenty. In our country bad nutrition is usually found among overweight or obese people. It is seldom a matter of emaciation. A high-fat, high-sugar diet is the surest road to malnutrition in America. It is also the easiest diet to get in your supermarket.

Gremlins Behind Degenerative Diseases

Not too many years ago, the reasons for the high rates of degenerative disease in the United States were not known. However, in the last 25 years a very large amount of effort has been put into studying the causes of the degenerative diseases, particularly the major degenerative diseases—heart disease and atherosclerosis. Today it is known that degenerative diseases in the United States are, to a large extent, caused by the kind of food we eat. Furthermore, the harmful ingredients in our food (which we shall call gremlins) have pretty much been identified. They include fat, cholesterol, sugar, salt, and caffeine.

FAT

Man has always eaten fat, but seldom in such large quantities as the modern American. While 42 percent of the calories of an average American diet are derived from fat, a primitive man probably received only 10 percent or less of his calories from fat. This is one reason why degenerative diseases are a plague to the modern American but are unknown to the primitive whose diet was a low-fat one. Although there is controversial evidence that large amounts of unsaturated fats such as safflower oil are better for you than large amounts of saturated fats such as animal fats, there is much evidence that *no* added fats are better than either saturated or unsaturated fats. Of all the multitude of fats found in nature, only one is necessary in your diet. It is the fat made from linoleic acid. It is called "essential" fat and it, or one of its near relatives, needs to be included in the food you eat. However, it is needed only in very small quantities. The 2100 Program diet will supply far more than the minimum levels of essential fat.

CHOLESTEROL

It was a surprise to many people that cholesterol should be one of the gremlins behind degenerative diseases. It was surprising because cholesterol is necessary for life, is produced throughout the body, and has many bodily uses. Cholesterol does its damage by causing the growth of mushy abscesses in the interior of the arteries. This condition, called atherosclerosis, is indirectly responsible for heart disease and stroke.

The atherosclerotic process can be reversed if the amount of cholesterol and fat in the blood is greatly reduced. Such a reduction is only possible if much less cholesterol is contained in the food we eat. Cholesterol in food is present in all animal products but is absent from all vegetable products. Low cholesterol diets stress low consumption of meats but allow all vegetables and fruits. The best way to see if the cholesterol gremlin is already a problem with you is to ask your doctor for a cholesterol check. If your cholesterol level is 150 or below, you are below normal, and in this country that is good. Your chances of having a heart attack, for example, are only a tenth what they would be if your level were 220—the American average.

SUGAR

Your body needs sugar to live. Sugar is burned by your body cells to generate the energy necessary to run the cell. But the sugar in your body is best obtained from the complex carbohydrates found in vegetables, bread, and the like.

Simple carbohydrates such as table sugar, honey, and molasses cause your body a great deal of difficulty. It is known that simple carbohydrates, or simple sugars as they are also called, raise the level of the blood fats, help to cause diabetes, and increase the cholesterol level in the blood.

SALT

One of the degenerative diseases is hypertension or high blood pressure. We know that the sodium in ordinary table salt is a cause of hypertension. Northern Japan, where great amounts of salt are used in food, has the highest incidence of hypertension in the world. In the United States it is often customary to salt everything: the cooking pot, the plate, and each bite. This level of dietary sodium paves the way to a case of hypertension and its complications.

CAFFEINE

We think of coffee or tea as being safe beverages: They may keep us awake at night, but they will not harm us. Today we know that the caffeine in coffee and tea gives us a jolt because it increases the free fatty acids in our bloodstream. We also know that continuous high levels of free fatty acids are likely to help in the development of atherosclerosis, diabetes, and heart disease.

Diet Types and Degenerative Disease

The foods you eat could be leading you down the path of degenerative disease. Find yourself on the chart which follows (Figure 6) and see. The numbers on the chart are approximations based on an elaboration of the diets shown, and are for men in their forties and fifties. But no matter what your age or sex, the *trend* of the chart is the same.

Figure 6.

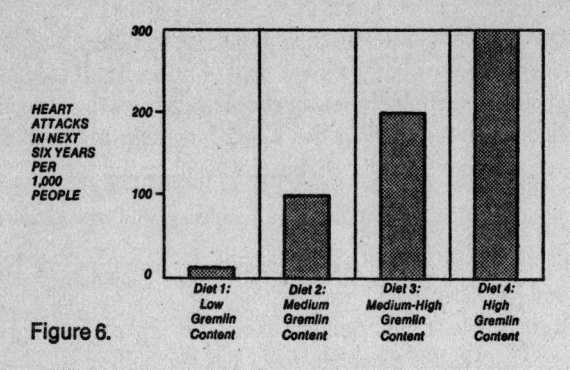

HEART ATTACKS IN NEXT SIX YEARS PER 1,000 PEOPLE

- Diet 1: Low Gremlin Content
- Diet 2: Medium Gremlin Content
- Diet 3: Medium-High Gremlin Content
- Diet 4: High Gremlin Content

Diet 1: 2100 Program foods.

Diet 2: Lean meats, low-fat cottage cheese and milk—sugary beverages and foods (including breads, and the like, made with sugar)—salt on food—caffeine in coffee and tea.

Diet 3: Lean meats, eggs, shellfish, cheeses, milk, organ meats (such as liver)—sugary foods and beverages—salt—caffeine.

Diet 4: Steak, sausage, bacon, eggs, shellfish, cheeses, milk, organ meats, and so forth—sugary food and beverages—salt—caffeine.

FIVE COMMANDMENTS FOR HEALTHY EATING

Nine of Moses' Ten Commandments are negative ones. Except for "Honor thy father and mother," they all begin with "Thou shalt not." So it is with the five commandments for healthy eating—they all begin with "Don't." They are negative commandments because they are addressing five food gremlins behind degenerative diseases. These gremlins can be thought of as poisons in our food, and for all poisons the best advice is negative: Don't eat them.

1. **DON'T EAT FATS OR OILS**
   Avoid fatty meats: Fatty hamburgers, fatty steak, and the like.
   Avoid oils: Cooking oils, salad oils, shortening.
   Avoid oily plants: Olives, avocadoes, nuts, and the like.
   Avoid: All dairy products except nonfat products.

2. **DON'T EAT SUGAR**
   Avoid: Sugar, honey, molasses, syrup, and so forth.
   Avoid: Pies, cakes, and pastries.
   Avoid: Breads, cereals, and the like which contain sugar.

3. **DON'T EAT SALT**[*]
   Don't: Salt your plate or the cooking pot.
   Avoid: Obviously salty products such as crackers and salted herring.

4. **DON'T EAT CHOLESTEROL**
   Limit: Your meat intake to 1/4 pound of lean meat per day.
   Avoid: Animal organs (brains, liver, and the like), animal skin, shellfish, eggs.

5. **DON'T DRINK COFFEE OR TEA**
   (You can drink tea made from herbs.)

---

[*] You cannot live without some fat and some salt. On the other hand even if you try very hard to avoid both, you will get plenty of each in your vegetables. For all practical purposes, therefore, you should follow the commandments just as they are written.

IS DIET REALLY IMPORTANT?

A Case History

Most people remember Dr. Philip Blaiberg, the South African dentist, at one time the longest surviving heart transplant patient. He died 19 months after his heart transplant, not of tissue rejection, as people thought at first, but of a heart attack. The doctor who examined Blaiberg's heart after he died found the heart's arteries choked with atherosclerosis. This same doctor had examined the new heart before the transplant and knew that the arteries were as clean as a baby's at that time.

During the entire 19 months with his new heart, Dr. Blaiberg maintained a high level of blood cholesterol. It started out at 315 and never dropped below 300. The kind of food that Blaiberg needed to drop his cholesterol level to a low value was never provided him. The diet that destroyed his first heart did just as effective a job destroying his second heart.

GETTING 2100 PROGRAM MEALS ONTO THE TABLE

The five commandments for healthy living form the basic ground rules for the things that should not be eaten, and the charts on the previous pages give us some ideas for what can be eaten. Already then we have begun to get some idea of what foods can be used and what foods should be avoided. A handy Use and Avoid List is presented as an appendix and also a longer list of basic foods that can be eaten within the 2100 Program limits. Therefore a diligent person should be able to find plenty of nutritious foods in the market that will conform to the 2100 requirements and that will provide him with variety. But that is a long way from getting 2100 Program meals onto the table. In the next few pages we shall discuss a few of the steps that will help to gear meal preparation the 2100 way.* The steps discussed will be:

* Throughout this chapter we are assuming that you will be wholeheartedly embracing the 2100 Eating Program. However, it is clear that this is very hard for many readers to do. In the last chapter of this book we therefore discuss how one may enter the program more gradually.

LIVE LONGER NOW

Your New Shopping List
Sample Menu for a Day
Planning 2100 Program Dinners
Tips for Cooking
Recipes for Delicious Dishes

Shopping List

What should you buy when you go to the store? The next few pages list many things that conform to the 2100 Food Program's five commandments. These pages should give you some ideas for what to buy the next time you go grocery shopping.

STAPLES
Unbleached or whole grain
  flours
Cornmeal
Cornstarch

Pancake mixes *
Tapioca
Knox gelatin
Vinegar

* You may be able to locate a brand free of such undesirables as sweeteners and additives.

COOKED CEREALS
Wheatena *
Cream of Wheat *
Roman Meal *

* These three supermarket cereals are the best of their kind, but be sure to get *regular* Cream of Wheat.

Rolled Oats and other **
  whole grains plain
  or in blends

** A good selection is often available in natural food stores.

DRY CEREALS
Grape Nuts *
Shredded Wheat *
Wheat, rye, and oat flakes

* Supermarket cereals are dreadful; these two are the best of a sad lot—though both contain additives. Health store cereals may be no better. Granola and other "natural" cereals have sweetening. In puffed cereals, the protein is damaged by steam used in the processing.

BREAD
Sourdough bread and rolls *

* Those made with only flour, water, salt. Avoid those containing shortening, sweeteners, or additives.

Part or 100 percent whole grain bread or rolls (whole wheat, rye, pumpernickel—plain or in blends) **

** It is not easy to locate whole or partially whole-grain breads without shortening, sweeteners, or additives. Some small bakers take large orders (20 loaves or more) which you can divide with friends or freeze.

SPECIALTY BREADS
Corn tortillas *

* Corn, lime, water. Flour tortillas, sadly, contain shortening.

Pita (Armenian) **   ** Flour, yeast, water, salt. These round flat yeast breads are great for "stuffing" sandwich-fashion. Try a foreign grocery if you don't find them elsewhere.

CRACKERS

Scandinavian type *   * Flour, water, salt (some varieties have skimmed milk). Avoid shortening, sweeteners and additives.

Matzoh **   ** Flour, water, salt. Some varieties have eggs and shortening—to be avoided!

DAIRY FOODS

Milk, skimmed (fresh, canned, dried) *   * Make sure it is nonfat, not low fat.

Eggs (whites only permissible)

Cheese, 100 percent skim milk varieties only (hoop, pot, baker's, farmer's) **   ** Some dairies deliver this kind of cheese. All other cheeses contain too much fat. Even low-fat cottage cheese is too high. Although its fat content by *weight* is 2 to 3 percent, the total *calories* in low-fat cottage cheese is 12 to 18 percent.

Buttermilk ••• ••• Most brands unacceptable due to too high fat content. Find kinds under 1 percent fat by weight, or use unhomogenized type from which fat particles can be sieved.

JUICES
Juices (canned or frozen) — Watch for sugar and additives, avoiding those products which contain them.

POULTRY, MEAT, FISH
Fish and shellfish (canned, fresh, or frozen) — Most shellfish are out due to high cholesterol content. Use water-packed canned fish only. Leaner fish varieties preferred (sole, halibut, snapper, etc.)

Poultry (fresh, frozen, or canned) — Chicken or turkey (especially the white meat) are best—avoid the skin. Duck, goose, and ground turkey are too fat.

Meat (fresh, frozen, or canned) — No marbled or fatty meats (spareribs, mutton, bacon, hot dogs, sausage, fatty hamburger, luncheon meats); no organ meats (liver, heart, kidney, sweetbreads).

DRIED FOODS
Rice (brown preferred)
Barley
Bulgur wheat *
Split peas
Lentils
Beans (many varieties: red, lima, pinto, kidney, navy, etc.)
Minced onion, parsley, bell peppers **
Spices, as desired ***

* Middle East rice substitute—cooks fast (15 minutes); good flavor and texture. (You may be able to locate it under brand name "Ala.")

** Come in packets or jars and are most handy.

*** Avoid premixed spice blends which contain sugar or additives.

PRODUCE
Vegetables (fresh, dried, canned, or frozen) *

Fruits (Fresh, dried, canned, or frozen) **

* Avoid avocado, olives, and all nuts, due to high fat content. Avoid canned vegetables with sugar or additives (corn and kidney beans usually have sugar); avoid frozen vegetables in sauces.

** Dried fruit should be restricted (no more than 2 oz. daily of larger fruits or 1 oz. raisins). Canned or frozen fruits—watch for sugar. Dietetic canned fruit without sugar substitutes or additives is fine.

SOUPS

Soups (canned, frozen, or dehydrated) *

* Acceptable soups are rare —most have fat and various additives, as do bouillon cubes. A good chicken broth (comes in jars) is Lynden's (Seattle, Wash.); Anderson's canned split pea soup is all right (but has monosodium glutamate, to which purists may object).

PASTAS *
Macaroni
Spaghetti

* Flour, water. Try the whole wheat pasta as a healthful change.

Noodles **

** Avoid egg or spinach noodles (which contain egg).

Planning Dinners

You need a workable strategy for your dinner plans to help you to accomplish your goal—producing delicious dinners without violating the 2100 Program commandments.

Start the meal with a hearty soup. A soup can be completely fat- and cholesterol-free while still satisfying your appetite. You can prepare soup in large batches, freezing quantities for future meals.

Routinely include a large salad of mixed lettuce combined with other vegetables, raw or cooked. (Try adding cooked pinto or garbonzo beans to a green salad. Delicious!) The salad helps fill your plate, satisfies the need to chew, and provides bulk and nourishment you need.

Serve several cooked vegetable and carbohydrate courses. Have one green and one yellow vegetable and at least one —maybe two—carbohydrate courses such as a 2100-style lasagna or spaghetti. The leftover vegetables and the liquids in which they were cooked can be used in the next night's soup or frozen for a future soup. Be sure to offer lots of bread with your meal, too.

The meat, poultry, or fish dish now has been removed from center stage to a position of lesser importance—thanks to putting more emphasis on other meal elements. For the meat, poultry, or fish dish, cultivate recipes in which these foods are used in combination with many other ingredients, such as stews or chop-suey-type dishes. You can "cheat" on the amounts of the meat, poultry, or fish, using smaller amounts in proportion to the other required ingredients. You will find even then that your dish is adequately flavored. Or, as a nice change you can substitute a vegetable entrée for the meat, poultry, or fish dish.

A practice that has several benefits is to cook up enough meat for several meals when using the leaner cuts that require long slow cooking and to freeze the surplus. The vegetables can be added later when the cooked meats in the freezer are taken out for future meals. This is a big time-saver. It also helps to reduce meat intake as you will find yourself "budgeting" each cut of meat for more than one meal.

Dessert, if desired, can be fruit or fruit salad, or you can prepare simple but satisfying specialties.

Sample Menu for a Day
This sample menu is just one of many that can be conceived. We picked it out to give you an idea of what a daily menu might look like. Feel free to invent menus that are the best and most appropriate for you and your family's own tastes.

BREAKFAST
Fruit: Oranges, Apples, and/or Strawberries
Whole Rolled Oatmeal * with Sliced Banana and Skim Milk
Tomato Juice
Sourdough Toast
Coffee (decaffeinated) with or without Skim Milk

LUNCH
Holiday Salad † with Buttermilk Spring Dressing †
Rice and Beans Steamed in Spices
Hoop Cheese Sandwiches on Rye ‡ with Lettuce and Tomatoes

DINNER
Mixed Green Salad
Briny Deep Salmon Loaf † or Enchiladas de Tijuana †
Acapulco Brown Rice †
Santa Barbara Split Pea Soup †
Sourdough Bread
Baked Potato with Mock Sour Cream † and Chives
Coffee (decaffeinated), Milk (skim), or Water

SNACKS BETWEEN MEALS
Fruit, Bread Slices (sourdough or acceptable rye), Crackers (unsalted, acceptable varieties), Beverages (acceptable varieties)

Tips for Cooking
Adopting a new way of eating entails freeing yourself from old habits of food preparation. A few suggestions are pro-

---

* One cup oatmeal with one cup water. Cook for two to three minutes, stirring constantly. Add banana slices before or after cooking.
† See Recipes for Delicious Dishes.
‡ Rye Bread containing no simple sugars, shortening, or additives.

vided to ease you into the new cooking style, but try your own innovations as you go. It can be fun. The nonstick cooking surfaces (teflon) will be most useful to you in baking and cooking in your new fat-free style of food preparation.

INGREDIENT SUBSTITUTIONS

Food can be prepared and many recipes can be made most successfully using minor ingredient substitutions. Here are some ideas:

OMIT	SUBSTITUTE
Whole milk	Use skim milk or other permissible liquid.*
Whole eggs	Use whites only, adding 1–2 tablespoons of permissible liquid to make up volume difference for each missing yolk. (Another good way is to use *two* egg whites—without yolks—for each egg required by the recipe.)
Oil or melted shortening	Adequate results can often be obtained by substituting an equal volume of permissible liquid.
Sugar, honey, and so forth	Use alone or in combinations to achieve desired sweetness: grated Delicious apple, cut-up or mashed bananas, a few raisins, frozen unsweetened fruit such as dark sweet cherries or blueberries and/or fruit juice, regular or frozen concentrated (undiluted or partially diluted).
Ricotta or cottage cheese	Mash hoop or other skim milk cheese with water or skim milk to achieve comparable texture. (Use in lasagna, manicotti, noodle kugel.)

* By permissible liquid we mean any liquid which does not violate the 2100 Program five commandments, such as skim milk, fruit juices, vegetable juices, herb and water mixtures, and so forth.

Sour cream — Place crumbled hoop or other skim milk cheese into blender, adding enough liquid (buttermilk, skim milk or water) to achieve texture approximating sour cream. Stir from time to time during blending. (Use over baked potatoes, fresh or frozen fruit, salads, in gelatin molds.)

SKIMMING FAT FROM COOKED DISHES

Many dishes can be refrigerated for a few hours or overnight (or even placed in freezer for a short period) to congeal fat for easy removal.

(If you lack the time to follow above procedure, try removing fat from liquid using a turkey baster.)

VEGETABLE SAUTÉING WITHOUT FAT

Place a little water in bottom of skillet, add vegetables and cook until done over moderate flame, stirring as needed. (Add a little extra water from time to time if vegetables become too dry during cooking process.) A second method is to place the chopped vegetables on a moderately hot teflon pan and cook until done, stirring as needed.

Try sautéing a large quantity of vegetables at one time; put them into freezer packets (plastic sandwich bags are fine) so they are ready for instant use in soups, stews, and the like.

MEAT BROWNING

Ground meat or meat with some visible fat can be browned directly—without adding fat, in a preheated heavy pan (or teflon utensil), as some fat will render from the meat in the cooking. As the meat sticks loosen it from bottom with a spatula and stir.

With leaner meats, slow-brown them starting with a cold teflon skillet, then add meat plus a tablespoon or two of liquid (water, broth, tomato juice), heating over a moderate flame and stirring occasionally. Continue heating until enough fat from meat has rendered into skillet and meat has become well-browned, after which onions, garlic, green pepper, and so on may also be added for browning. The process takes a bit of time but results are good.

Another method is to place meat under the broiler for quick browning, then removing from broiler to continue preparation on top of stove or in oven. The method works well with such foods as pot roasts, stew meat, and chicken. (When used with chicken, strip the skin from all of the pieces before placing on broiler pan.) Baste if required with rendered juices.

BREADING CHICKEN, FISH, VEAL, EGGPLANT, ETC.

Step 1. Moisten each piece in suitable liquid—skim milk, water, chicken broth, tomato juice or purée. (For chicken, remove skin first.)

Step 2. Dip in breading mixture (seasoned cornmeal, matzoh meal, flour, dry bread crumbs, or cereal). Place on teflon baking surface and bake in preheated moderate oven. Baste with liquid if desired. (Veal may require covering for first part of cooking period to tenderize properly.)

RECIPES FOR DELICIOUS DISHES

On the following pages we have collected recipes * for delicious dishes. These dishes are some of the favorites of people in the Longevity Foundation. To a great extent they are simple modifications of long-time family recipes, in which

---

* These recipes occasionally call for packaged or canned foods as ingredients; it is important to read the labels on what you buy, and buy only those brands the contents of which do not violate the 2100 Program's five commandments.

substitutions and allowances for nonacceptable ** ingredients have been made. You will find them delightful.

Salads

BASIC INGREDIENT SUGGESTIONS:

GREENS

lettuce (all types), celery, spinach, kale, chicory, watercress, endive, romaine, fennel, green cabbage, red cabbage, escarole, collards, swiss chard, arugula, comfrey, sorrel, vegetable tops, green onions, scallions, shallots, broccoli leaves, young green peas

HERBS

parsley, mint, oregano, sage, garlic, tarragon, basil, dill, chervil, chives, thyme, savory, marjoram, rosemary

OTHER INGREDIENTS

tomatoes (all types), cucumbers, sweet green or red peppers, radishes, steamed string beans (cooled), cooked artichoke hearts (cooled), 100 percent skim milk cheese, raw peas, raw beets, raw young asparagus tips, onions, parsnip, hardcooked egg white, cooked potatoes (cooled), carrots, fruit

** "Nonacceptable" means not complying with the 2100 Program's five commandments.

HOLIDAY SALAD: *Serves 6*

¾ cup asparagus tips, steamed
¾ cup string beans, steamed
¾ cup cucumbers, diced
½ cup young peas, raw
½ cup radishes, sliced
2 artichoke hearts, cooked and sliced
2 egg whites, hard cooked and sliced

Toss all ingredients lightly. Moisten with Buttermilk Spring Dressing.

RAINY DAY SALAD: *Serves 6*

1 cup beets, cooked and diced
1 cup potatoes, cooked and diced
½ cup diced apple with skin
1 green pepper and 1 stalk celery, diced

Toss all ingredients lightly. Moisten with remaining beet juice for tint. Add Buttermilk Spring Dressing.

BUTTERMILK SPRING DRESSING

1 cup buttermilk *
1 tsp. frozen apple juice (concentrate)
1 tsp. lemon juice
1 tsp. dried onion flakes
1 tsp. dill weed

Season to taste with pepper and ground allspice. Mix all ingredients. Chill.

* Use unhomogenized buttermilk, and strain to remove butterfat particles.

AUTUMN BEAN DRESSING

1 16 oz. can cooked red or pinto beans, undrained
2 tbsp. cider or wine vinegar
¼ cup apple or pineapple juice
½ tsp. onion flakes
½ tsp. dill weed or basil
Pepper to taste

Mix all ingredients, including liquid from canned beans. Chill.

MOCK SOUR CREAM

Put quantity of crumbled hoop cheese ** into blender. Blend with sufficient liquid (buttermilk,* skim milk, water) to achieve consistency of sour cream. Stir contents as needed during blending. Excellent on salads, baked potatoes, and the like.

Hearty Soups

GREEK LENTIL SOUP: *Serves 6*

1 cup lentils
1 med. onion, chopped
1 stalk celery, chopped
1 bay leaf
¼ tsp. oregano
2 tbsp. wine vinegar
3 tbsp. tomato paste
2 qts. liquid—chicken broth or water, or some of both

** Hoop cheese is made from 100 percent nonfat milk. Synonyms sometimes used are: Farmer's cheese, baker's cheese, and pot cheese.

Wash and drain lentils. Put all ingredients except wine vinegar into soup pot; bring to boil and simmer covered for about 1½ hours or until lentils are very soft, stirring occasionally if needed. Add wine vinegar. Purée about half the mixture in food mill or blender; return puréed mixture, combining with balance in pot. Stir, heat and serve.

SANTA BARBARA SPLIT PEA SOUP: *Serves 6*

1¼ cups green or yellow split peas
1 med. onion, chopped
1 stalk celery, chopped
2 carrots, diced
½ tsp. marjoram

⅛ tsp. ground cloves
2 qts. liquid—chicken broth or water, or some of both (use less liquid for a thicker soup)

Wash and drain peas. Put all ingredients into soup pot; bring to boil and simmer, covered, for about 1½ hours or until peas are mushy, stirring occasionally if needed. Purée about half the mixture in food mill or blender; return puréed mixture, combining with balance in pot. Stir, heat, and serve.

GAZPACHO (SPANISH SALAD SOUP): *Serves 8*

1 cucumber, peeled and finely chopped
6 large ripe tomatoes, peeled and finely chopped
2 cloves garlic, minced
1 small green pepper, finely chopped
2 celery stalks, finely chopped
8 green onions, finely chopped

1 handful parsley, finely chopped
2 tbsp. wine vinegar
½ tsp. dill
¼ tsp. thyme
¼ tsp. mint
Thin slices lemon for garnish
5 cups liquid (3 cups chicken broth, 2 cups tomato juice)

To peel tomatoes, scald quickly in very hot water. Combine all ingredients, stir well. Purée half the mixture in food mill or blender; combine with balance. Cover. Chill overnight or longer. Add water to thin, if desired. Stir well before serving. Garnish bowls or mugs with lemon.

MINESTRONE: Serves 6–8

- 1 med. onion, chopped
- 1 clove garlic, minced
- 1 leek, diced (when available)
- 2 tbsp. chopped parsley
- ½ tsp. thyme
- ½ tsp. oregano
- 3 tbsp. tomato paste
- 1 large can (28 oz.) tomatoes, chopped
- 3 stalks celery, chopped
- 2 carrots, diced
- 2 cups shredded cabbage
- 2 zucchini, diced
- ⅓ cup uncooked brown rice
- 3 cups cooked dried beans
- 1½ qts. liquid—chicken broth, water, or some of both

Put all ingredients except rice and beans into soup pot; bring to boil, add rice, then simmer, covered, for 1 hour. Now add beans. Purée a portion (about ⅓) of mixture in food mill or blender; return puréed mixture, combining with balance in pot. Stir, heat, and serve.

CABBAGE/BEET BORSCHT: *Serves 6*

4–5 cups shredded cabbage
1 med. onion, chopped
1 large can (28 oz.) tomatoes, finely chopped
1 16 oz. can beets, coarsely chopped
4 oz. apple juice
1/8 tsp. nutmeg
2 cups water

Put all ingredients into soup pot; bring to boil. Simmer, covered, for about 40 minutes. Thin with water, if desired. Serve hot.

FRESH FROZEN PEA * SOUP: *Serves 4*

4 cups frozen peas
1 tbsp. dried onion
Pepper to taste
1 cup liquid—water or skim milk

Put peas, dried onion, and liquid of choice into soup pot and bring to boil. Simmer, covered, until vegetables are tender. Put entire mixture through blender (start blender at medium, then go to high speed). Return contents to pot, seasoning with pepper, if desired. Thin with additional water or milk, if desired. Serve hot.

* Corn, in same quantity, may be substituted for the peas to make a corn soup.

Italian Entrées

SPAGHETTI

TWO MARINARA SAUCES

I: Serves 4

1 large can (28 oz.) Italian plum tomatoes, finely chopped	1 tsp. oregano ¼ cup chopped parsley 1 clove garlic, finely minced

Cook rapidly, uncovered, about 15 minutes or until thickened, stirring occasionally. If sauce becomes too thick, add ¼ to ½ cup water. Serve hot on spaghetti.

II: Serves 4

1 med. onion, finely chopped 1 clove garlic, finely minced 2 16-oz. cans Italian plum tomatoes, finely chopped	½ tsp. basil ¼ tsp. thyme ¼ tsp. parsley

Bring a small quantity (about 4 oz.) water to boil in skillet. Add onion and garlic and cook over moderate flame until tender and slightly yellowed. Add remaining ingredients. Simmer over low heat for 15–20 minutes. Serve hot on spaghetti.

MANICOTTI OR LASAGNA: *Serves 5*

Mash 3 cups of hoop cheese with three egg whites, 2 tsp. dried parsley, and enough water to achieve a consistency like that of cottage cheese.

Boil lasagna or manicotti noodles to "al dente" stage (not too well done); pour off water and set noodles in cool water while preparing casserole.

FOR MANICOTTI: Stuff each drained noodle with hoop cheese mixture, using long-handled teaspoon to fill. Lay the noodles in baking dish over thin layer of Marinara sauce. Cover with generous layer of Marinara sauce. Bake in 375° oven for approximately 30 minutes or until slightly browned on top.

FOR LASAGNA: Place a thin layer of Marinara sauce on bottom of rectangular baking dish, then place a layer of drained noodles over this, then a layer of hoop cheese mixture, then sauce. Repeat this sequence, building up several noodle layers. End with sauce. Bake in 375° oven for about 45 minutes or until slightly browned on top.

VENICE COMBINATION PIZZA: *Serves 4–6*
(*Recipe for two pizzas*)

DOUGH:
1. Soften ½ pkg. (1 tsp.) active dry yeast in 2 tbsp. warm water (110–115° F.). Let stand 5–10 minutes.
2. Meanwhile, pour into large bowl 1 cup warm water. Blend in 2 cups sifted flour. Stir softened yeast; add to flour-water mixture, mixing well.
3. Measure 2 cups sifted flour. Add about ½ the flour to yeast mixture; beat until very smooth. Mix in enough remaining flour to make a soft dough. Turn mixture onto a lightly floured surface. Allow to rest 5–10 minutes. Knead.
4. Select a deep bowl just large enough to allow dough to double. Shape dough into smooth ball and place in very lightly greased bowl. Turn dough to bring greased sur-

face to top. Cover with waxed paper (or plastic wrap) and towel and place in warm place (about 80° F.) until dough is doubled (about 1½ to 2 hours).
5. Punch down with fist. Fold edge toward center and turn dough over. Divide dough into two equal balls. Grease a second bowl. Place each ball of dough into a greased bowl. Turn greased side up. Cover as before. Let rise again until almost double (about 45 minutes).
6. Roll each ball of dough into a round to fit 14" pizza pan which has been greased (unless teflon) or into a 10" x 14" rectangle to fit rectangular pan. Shape edge of pizzas by pressing dough between thumb and forefinger to make ridge.

TOPPING:

- 1 small can tomato paste
- 1 med. onion, chopped
- ⅔ green pepper, chopped
- ½ lb. extra lean ground beef, crumbled
- 2 cups crumbled hoop cheese
- 1 small can drained sliced mushrooms
- 4 tsp. oregano
- 2 cloves garlic, finely minced

COOKING:

1. Divide the topping ingredients and sprinkle over each pizza, in order of listing.
2. Bake at 400° F. approximately 25 minutes, or until slightly browned on top.

Sea Food Entrées

BRINY DEEP SALMON LOAF: *Serves 4*

LOAF INGREDIENTS:

1 8-oz. can salmon	½ cup skim milk
3 cups soft bread crumbs (sourdough bread crumbs are fine)	½ cup chopped onion
	2 tbsp. chopped parsley
	½ tsp. tarragon
3 egg whites	

Drain salmon, and remove skin and bones. Combine loaf ingredients, mixing and mashing well to distribute salmon, wet ingredients, and seasonings thoroughly in bread crumbs. Shape and place mixture in an 8" x 8" x 2" teflon pan and bake in preheated 400° F. oven for 20–25 minutes or until done.

Sauce ingredients:

1¾ cups frozen peas	1 tsp. curry powder
2 tbsp. chopped pimiento	½ tsp. tarragon
1 cup milk	2 tbsp. cornstarch

To prepare sauce layer, cook 1¾ cups frozen peas in small amount of water until done. Add chopped pimiento and milk and heat until mixture begins to boil. Mix 2 tbsp. of water with the cornstarch and curry powder in small bowl and add this to the pea mixture, stirring and cooking over low heat until liquid thickens. Layer the curried pea mixture over entire surface of salmon loaf and serve.

NEPTUNE'S CHOWDER: *Serves 8*

- 1 stalk celery, chopped
- 1 med. onion, chopped
- 1 leek, chopped (when available)
- 1 clove garlic, finely minced
- 1 large carrot, diced
- 2 tbsp. chopped parsley
- 1 can (28 oz.) tomatoes, chopped
- 1 small can (8 oz.) tomato sauce
- 2 bay leaves
- ¾ tsp. thyme
- Pepper to taste
- ¾ cup sherry wine
- 2 cups water
- 3 large cooked potatoes, peeled and diced
- 1 lb. fish fillets (red snapper, sea bass, halibut, or other firm-fleshed fish) cut in 1½" squares
- Juice of 1 lemon
- 3 tbsp. cornstarch mixed with a few tbsp. water

Bring small quantity of water (about 4 oz.) to boil in soup pot; add celery, onion, leek, and garlic and cook until vegetables are tender and slightly yellowed. Add carrots, tomatoes, tomato sauce, parsley, bay leaves, thyme, and water and bring to boil. Simmer slowly covered for about 30 minutes.

Add wine, lemon juice, fish, and potatoes and simmer slowly covered for another 20 minutes. Add pepper to taste, if desired.

Add cornstarch mixed with few tablespoons of water, stirring into contents to thicken. Let cook another few minutes.

Specialty Entrées

CHICKEN FRICASSEE WITH VEGETABLES AND DUMPLINGS: *Serves 4*

½ broiler-fryer, cut-up, completely skinned
3⅓ cups chicken broth or water
1 med. onion, chopped
1 stalk celery, diced
1 bay leaf
½ tsp. turmeric powder

1 small cabbage, cut in eighths
8 small onions, peeled
4 carrots, pared and cut in 2–3" chunks
1 cup frozen peas
4 tbsp. flour blended with ½ cup cold water

DUMPLING BATTER:
2 cups flour
4 tsp. baking powder
2 tsp. finely minced parsley

1 scant cup skim milk

Completely remove fat from chicken. Put chicken in kettle, add broth or water, chopped onion and celery, and turmeric and bay leaf. Bring to boil; simmer, covered, for 30 minutes or until chicken is almost tender. Skim any fat that appears in broth. Now add carrots, cabbage, and onions; simmer, covered, for another 20 minutes. Mix in peas, let simmering begin again, then stir in the flour which has been blended with water, mixing well. Quickly add dumpling batter * by teaspoonfuls onto simmering surface, spacing droppings apart, cover tightly, and steam 10 minutes without lifting lid. Remove lid, turn dumplings over to moisten dry side. Serve with turmeric rice (cook rice with ½ tsp. turmeric per cup of raw rice, using combination of about ⅓ chicken broth, ⅔ water for cooking liquid).

TO MAKE DUMPLINGS:

Put flour and baking powder through sifter once to blend. Add minced parsley and skim milk, stirring to moisten all of flour mixture. Drop onto simmering stew as directed.

MOUSSAKA: *Serves 4*
(Ground beef and eggplant in a Greek specialty) *

1 large eggplant (or 2 smaller ones)	¼ cup red wine
½ lb. extra-lean ground beef	½ tsp. cinnamon
	¼ tsp. nutmeg
1 med. onion, chopped	2 tbsp. chopped parsley
1 clove garlic, minced	1 egg white
1 can (8 oz.) tomato sauce	1 tbsp. flour mixed with 2 tbsp. water

1. Slice eggplant crosswise in pieces about ½" thick. Lay on teflon baking pan (or on foil-covered baking pan) and bake in hot oven (425° F.) until slightly browned. Turn slices to brown slightly on other side.
2. Meanwhile, brown ground beef directly in skillet, stirring constantly. Add onion and garlic and continue cooking and stirring over moderate flame. Add tomato sauce, wine, cinnamon, nutmeg, and parsley; let simmer for about 5 minutes.
3. Stir egg white into mixture of flour and water in small bowl, then add to simmering meat mixture, stirring until contents become thickened evenly.
4. Make layer of eggplant slices in large shallow baking pan, placing slices as close together as possible. Layer ground beef mixture evenly over eggplant slices (it will be a thin layer). Place in preheated oven and bake at 350° F. for approximately 30 minutes, or until top is slightly browned and casserole looks a little dry at edges.

* It you can find Armenian bread (pita), it is great to serve the bread warmed and to slip some of the Moussaka into it sandwich fashion. Rice or bulgur wheat is a good accompaniment, as is mock sour cream (*see* Salad Dressings).

FARMERS' ONION-CHEESE PIE: *Serves 4; 6 as side dish*

4 egg whites
1 cup hoop cheese
1 cup skim milk
6 tbsp. dried parsley

½ cup diced onions
1 tsp. prepared hot mustard
⅛ tsp. garlic powder

GARNISH:
2 tbsp. chopped pimiento
1½ tsp. dried onion

Put all ingredients except garnish into blender; blend at high speed until mixture becomes creamy. Pour into an 8" teflon pie pan. Place in preheated 325° F. oven and bake for one hour until crust is nicely browned. Put garnish on top after pie is about half baked.

Entrées from South of the Border

ENCHILADAS DE TIJUANA: *Serves 6*
(Turkey and bean)

1½ cups cooked kidney, pinto or red beans, drained well
2 cups diced cooked turkey *
2 small onions, finely chopped
1 clove garlic, minced
½ green pepper, finely chopped

1 tsp. oregano
2 oz. diced, canned green chiles (or canned whole green chiles, seeded and finely chopped)
3 cans (8 oz.) tomato sauce
12 corn tortillas
Green onion for garnish

* Cooked chicken or beef may be used instead of turkey.

Combine turkey and well-drained beans. Mash down beans and turkey (using fork or potato masher) so that they adhere to each other. Mix in half the chopped onion. Set mixture aside while preparing sauce.

Sauce: Bring a small quantity (about 4 oz.) of water to boil in skillet. Add green pepper, garlic, and rest of onion and cook over moderate flame until tender and slightly yellowed. Add tomato sauce, chiles, and oregano and simmer about 5 minutes.

Dip tortillas one by one in simmering sauce, filling each with turkey-bean-onion mixture, then rolling up and placing seam side down in shallow baking dish. Pour sauce over enchiladas. Bake at 350° for 20–25 minutes or until heated through. Garnish with chopped green onion. Serve with Acapulco brown rice.

ACAPULCO BROWN RICE

2 med. onions, chopped
1 clove garlic, minced
2 cups uncooked brown rice
2 cups water or chicken broth
1 cup tomato purée
1 tbsp. minced parsley

Heat heavy skillet over moderate flame and add rice, stirring frequently to toast rice lightly. Meanwhile bring water or chicken broth and purée to boil in separate container, then carefully pour all of liquid mixture over rice. Mix in onion, garlic, and parsley. Cover and turn heat down very low; let cook without lifting cover for about 40 minutes or until all of liquid is absorbed.

SOME EXTRA BENEFITS

A Heightening of Taste

Food needs to be delicious. Whatever else we say about the nutritional benefits of food, it should also be delightfully delicious to eat. And as simple and homely as the 2100 Program foods might at first seem to the gourmet, there is an incredible variety of taste sensations available among them. This is especially true after your taste buds have had a chance to adapt themselves to the light and airy flavors of 2100 Program foods. It is amazing how many delicious and subtle tastes are masked by the strong effects of salt, fat, and sugar. Although these great taste-maskers are everywhere evident in the American diet, they are not a part of the 2100 Program, and their absence will give you a chance to discover tastes you never knew existed.

A few weeks after you have started the program, you can expect to find that your tastes have changed so much that the thought of a pastry would hold little allure. In fact after this length of time, you would probably find that a high-sugar/high-fat American meal would cause you some discomfort. Your taste and your body will be tuned to a new wave length. Does this seem incredible to you? Try it, and see for yourself.

Sleep

Nearly everyone has from time to time had problems associated with sleep or sleepiness. Sometimes we find it hard to go to sleep even though we feel very much as though we need it; other times we find it hard to stay awake even though we would very much like to. For the insomniac the problem of sleeping can become a horrible nightmare of sleepiness and ineffectivity during daytime hours and sleeplessness during nighttime hours. For most of us it is simply a nuisance of varying degrees of irritation. But to all of us the

2100 Food Program is a blessing: It makes sleep easier to get when we want it and yet easier to avoid when we want to stay awake.

After a typically American, high-fat meal, it is common to feel drowsy. The reason for this is that the fat we have eaten is actually entering our bloodstream, lowering its oxygen-carrying capacity, and thereby dulling our minds and senses. In fact, on standard American diets high levels of fat are usually present in the blood all the time. By the same token the inability to turn off a tired, taut body at night and fall into a restful sleep may also be a product of diet. It seems to stem primarily from the nerve-jangling, free fatty acids that our standard eating habits keep constantly in our blood. The 2100 Food Program has the effect of keeping both fats and free fatty acids at very low levels in the blood. As a result sleepiness is slower to come when you do not want it; on the other hand the blessings of sleep are easier to find when you need them.

Weight

A person's weight is controlled by his appestat just as the temperature in a room is controlled by a thermostat. The mechanism by which the appestat works is a complex and little understood one involving both psychological and physical phenomena. But when it becomes maladjusted to the high side, for any reason, weight will be gained. Weight reduction diets rarely work over the long haul because, with a few exceptions, they seldom do anything to readjust the appestat. So the person who loses 10 pounds on a diet will usually put it all back on again and more within a few months.

The 2100 Food Program has a way of permanently readjusting the maladjusted appestat for the better. Food in the

2100 Program is so low in fats and simple sugars * that an overweight person may find that his appestat does not respond in its usual way. His appestat is apparently not prepared for foods lacking sugars and fats and will not readily call for more of them after a meal. By the time most people have adjusted to the 2100 Food Program, their appestats have sought and found a lower setting. It should be noted that thus far the experience in the Longevity Foundation seems to indicate that it is difficult to get fat on 2100 Program foods. (On the other hand maintenance of body weight has been no problem either.)

On the 2100 Food Program it is likely that you can stop calorie counting to control your weight. You can probably eat whatever you like and let your appestat control your weight for you. The calorie counting tables and the weight tables that you will find in other books on nutrition and dieting are not included in this book. They truly seem not to be necessary when the appestat is properly set.

Between-meal Endurance

One surprising aspect to the 2100 Food Program is that you do not get a between-meal letdown or rush of hunger that happens so often on the ordinary American diet. On the standard high-fat diet there is a need in most people to eat every four or five hours or else face a surge of irritability and depression that is caused by a between-meal falling blood sugar. This falling blood sugar seems to be completely a function of diet and appears to disappear altogether on the 2100 Food Program. You can go as long as you like between meals, and all you'll be is hungry. You are not

---

* Primitive societies on their native diets appear to have almost no problem with weight control. In some cases this may be due to a short supply of food, but even in cases in which calories abound, overweight appears to be rare. It is interesting to note that most primitive societies have an extreme low-fat/low-simple-sugar diet.

likely to get the dizzy, irritable, and depressed feeling that characterizes normal eating habits. Conversely, you can eat all you want on 2100 Program foods and still not get the bloated, overfilled feeling that is so disabling after a normal American meal.

Costs of Foods

Believe it or not, the 2100 Food Program is a relatively inexpensive way to eat. We estimate that your food costs will go down by about 30 percent if you are an average shopper. Your vegetable and fruit bills will go up slightly but your meat bills will go down drastically. The money you now spend on what we call the "garbage foods" such as children's breakfast cereals, potato chips, and so forth will be completely saved. All in all, even if you really let yourself go wild on fruits and vegetables, you will realize significant savings. Vegetables can stretch a dollar a long, long way.

CHAPTER 8

The 2100 Exercise Program

> Every adult should find time in his daily schedule for some form of physical activity. Medical evidence tells us that our hearts, lungs, muscles, and even our minds need the effects of regular vigorous exercise.
>
> Despite the comfort of modern existence, life still demands the best that we can give. Leisure must not mean physical inactivity and idleness. Instead we must recognize it as an opportunity to strengthen and refresh ourselves for our role as creative and productive citizens.
>
> From *Adult Physical Fitness* by the President's Council on Physical Fitness.

Everybody needs exercise. Exercise is the master conditioner of the healthy and a major therapy of the ill. It is a key element of long life, and it is a key protective element against disease.

Regular exercise helps to prevent and apparently to reverse degenerative diseases. Heart disease, the nation's number one killer, can be significantly alleviated by a suitable exercise program. Diabetes, a disease most people believe to be incurable, can often be prevented and reversed by the proper exercise program together with the proper food program. Atherosclerosis, stroke, and even gout can be overcome with exercise, combined with proper food.

The severity of many specific diseases that afflict people can be greatly reduced by regular exercise. But there is more to exercise than its disease-stopping power. It is also a way to make your life easier and brighter. A regular exercise program builds strength and endurance into your body so that every activity you encounter becomes easier. This is true for all activities—those on the job, at home, or those that are just for fun.

You look better and feel better when you exercise regularly. Not only does exercise help prevent disease and give you extra strength for your activities, it improves your posture, your complexion, and the shape of your body. Besides feeling better because you are indeed healthier, you also feel better because you know your looks have improved.

YOUR EXERCISE PROGRAM: ITS AIMS AND ITS POTENTIALS

To look your best, feel your best, and be resistant to heart disease and other degenerative diseases you need a program of exercise and activity. The aim of the 2100 Exercise Program is to provide you with this exercise and activity in the most natural and productive way possible. Your 2100 Exercise Program revolves around some basic facts about the human animal and his capabilities.

We all know that man has a powerful brain, but we tend to forget that man also has a body with great physical strength and endurance. We often think of the horse as the supreme animal for the speedy traveling of long distances. Yet according to the *Guinness Book of World Records* (1973), it is man that appears to hold all the truly impressive records for speedy long-distance travel on foot. In 1836 Mensen Ernst of Norway, traveling an average of 94 miles per day, covered a distance of more than 5,500 miles on foot in less than two months. Other examples of men covering thousands of miles on foot at such high rates are also mentioned in *Guinness*, yet only one record of a horse accomplishing an equivalent feat is recorded, the horse having covered some 1,200 miles in Portugal at some apparently unknown date in history and at some unknown rate.

At shorter distances the horse does a little better. According to *Guinness*, the horse Champion Crabbet is the holder of the world's record for long-distance racing and speed, having covered 300 miles at an average speed of 5.7 mph in 1920. On the other hand *Guinness* lists Wally Hayward as holding the human 24-hour running record, having covered 159 miles at an average speed of 6.7 mph. This was accomplished in 1954 when Wally was 45 years old. At very short distances, a few miles, a horse is far superior to man, running the mile, for example, in a little more than a minute and a half, compared to man's leisurely pace of four minutes.

But the point is, in addition to his superior brain power, man is also a very superior animal in his physical capacities. This seems to be particularly true for his ability to get around on foot, as the citations from *Guinness* amply illustrate.

Other than certain birds, man is the only animal that travels, both slow and fast, on two legs. He has a graceful striding gait that will carry him equally well at a snail's pace or a sprinter's. Fossil evidence has recently shown that man developed his unique striding form of locomotion more than a million years ago. The way we get around on two legs today is thus the same as the way we have moved ourselves for a million years. Perhaps it is this historical antiquity that makes walking and running such perfect sources of conditioning for the human body.

As we shall soon see in the paragraphs below, your 2100 Exercise Program capitalizes on the human being's unique and long-standing skill at two-legged locomotion; for this reason, it is particularly appropriate physiologically.

In addition to physiological considerations, your exercise program must be something that fits into your daily life, no matter what your situation might be. Whether you are a working person, a student, or a housewife, and regardless of your daily schedule or your daily mode of dress, the exercise program must be convenient for you to do. Then too, your exercise program must be fun. If it is not fun, more fun than other things you could be doing with your free time, then eventually you will stop doing it.

The 2100 Exercise Program is all of these things. It is physiologically appropriate, adaptable to any situation, and fun. The program revolves around a concept called "roving."

Roving: A Natural Exercise That Gives You the Most Return for Your Investment

Roving is a combination of walking and running with you in the pilot's seat. You decide if and when to run or whether merely to walk. Roving is the most natural of all exercises and has an extremely high-conditioning potential.

The key idea in roving is to set yourself a distance goal of so many miles. Then four or five times each week you set out to walk (or run if you prefer) that distance. Enjoy yourself as you go. Go different places on different days if you like. Change the scenery whenever you want to.

The central principle in roving is to cover a lot of ground, but to do it in your own good time. Roving can fit easily into the life of the average man or woman because it is so flexible. The working person can arrange to walk all or a part of the way to work each day. Daily excursions to the market, the park, or around the countryside are all good roving candidates.

Roving can start off as walking by itself, with no running at all. It may remain that way indefinitely. If it is at all possible, you should arrange your roving so that you can run during a rove whenever you feel like it. Physically it is beneficial, and it is very good emotionally to let a walking rove turn into a run then back into a walk, whenever you feel the urge. And you will feel the urge, once you have done it a few times. It is your million years of heredity coming into play that brings upon you a strong urge to lean forward and jog or run in the middle of a rove. If you have arranged things so that you can satisfy this urge without feeling foolish, it will be of great benefit to you. Arranging things so that you will not feel foolish usually means making sure your rove takes you through a large park or into the countryside, and making sure that the way you are dressed is appropriate for running as well as walking.

That is all there is to roving. Set your distance. Travel that distance on foot four or five times each week. Go for distance, not time. Allow yourself to satisfy the urge to run.

Exercise Program:
The Ten Fundamental Principles of Exercise
Utilizing the Concept of Roving

1. Distance is important; time is not.
2. Select a distance suited to yourself.
3. Rove your distance four or five times per week.
4. As warm-up, begin each rove at a slow pace. That is all the warm-up needed.
5. Increase your roving distance only when you are ready.
6. Use your heart recovery test as your gauge to slow down or speed up.
7. Give yourself variety.
8. Do not strain or compete against the clock or against people.
9. Always enjoy your roving.
10. The program is for everyone: young or old, male or female.

Easy? The above is the only exercise listing you will ever see in the 2100 Exercise Program. This is all there is to it.

The 2100 Exercise Program

Rules for Selecting Your Distance:
1. A few blocks if you are or have been very ill.
2. 1½ miles if you are healthy but in poor to average condition.
3. 3 miles if you are healthy and in good condition.
4. 6 to 10 miles if you are healthy and in excellent condition.

Heart Recovery Test *
1. After a rove, stop and rest 60 seconds.
2. Count your pulse (by feeling your wrist or your throat) over a 30-second time period.
3. If this 30-second count exceeds 65, slow down on subsequent roves.
4. When you are fully conditioned your 30-second count will be near 50, even under conditions of heavy exercise.

For Variety:
1. Change your path or schedule.
2. Try hills or a running track.
3. Rove with a friend or a group.

You Are Ready to Increase Your Roving Distance Only When:
1. You feel that you *can* rove the added distance.
2. You feel that you will *enjoy* the additional roving.
3. Your Heart Recovery Test gives a count of less than 65.

You Are Now Ready to Go
The fundamental principles described on the previous pages are all you need to know to get started on your 2100 Exercise Program. You can start today if it is not raining outside. Select your distance, figure out how to fit a little roving conveniently into your schedule, look around for some roving

---

* An adaptation of the internationally used Harvard Step Test.

routes, and you are in business. Do not be too particular about roving routes or what you wear to begin with. The most important thing is to get started. Good luck!

Shooting for High Levels of Physical Conditioning

Not everyone will want to shoot for high performance, at least at the outset. It is perfectly acceptable to achieve and maintain any roving distance that feels right to you. You do not have to feel that benefit will only come at high levels of conditioning. Even if you do not want to shoot for high performance right now, however, you should read these words on how to achieve high performance. Some principles are illustrated that are useful at all levels.

The trick with a high level of physical conditioning is to select a long roving distance. Suppose you select 10 miles. Although 10 miles is indeed a long distance, nearly anyone can cover it if he gives himself enough time. And in roving you always have plenty of time. The easiest and quickest way to cover 10 miles is to jog the distance at a speed that is comfortable to you.

The first few times you cover 10 miles it may be easy for you to hold your speed down. But soon your body will want to run faster than the pace you have set for it. Your body's strength will be growing, and you will probably find it difficult to keep your speed as low as in the beginning. You will naturally go faster. Gradually over the weeks, the length of time it takes you to cover 10 miles will grow shorter and shorter.

Several things should be noticed about achieving a high level of performance. First of all, it is almost necessary that you be able to jog or run during your roves. It is possible to walk your way to such a performance level, but somewhat difficult in practice.

Second, you need to be able to devote more than an hour for each rove. This is a lot of time, and it may be beyond the reach of many people. But if you can scrape up the time, the benefits to you are tremendous.

Lastly, we should note that for roves as long as 10 miles, you really do not need to rove four or five times every week. Three roves are ample. The one or two extra days per week that you pick up should be used for shorter roves or some other activity such as bicycling or swimming.

Remember, roving needs to be fun or it will not stay with you. Just because you are shooting for high performance does not mean that roving should be hard work for you. If it becomes hard work, you should switch back to a shorter roving distance. And if you find that you must switch back to a shorter distance, you need not feel defeated. Your goal should not focus on "world endurance records" or anything like that but simply on enjoying your roving. The only time you should feel defeated is when you can honestly say: "I am not enjoying what I am doing." That is the defeat, not the switch to a shorter distance.

Caution

If you are more than 30 the probability is very high that you have some amount of atherosclerosis. Even a little overexertion can lead to a fatal heart attack if you have severe atherosclerosis of the coronary arteries. It is therefore vital that your roving start slowly at a walking pace, and that you only increase your pace when you can do so without raising your heartbeat to more than 170 counts per minute while walking or running.

If you have reason to suspect that any exertion may cause your heart, joints, or other parts of your body some permanent damage, then you should consult your doctor before taking on the 2100 Exercise Program. Show him a copy of this book, and let him prescribe your roving for you.

Major Physiological Benefits of the 2100 Program

In conditioning your body, roving does a number of specific things. One of the most important is to increase the efficiency by which your body delivers oxygen to its various tissues. Oxygen delivery is improved in a number of ways. Brand new circulation is actually developed due to roving, with the growth of new capillaries to carry more blood to the body's muscles. This new circulation, called *collateral* circulation, enables the heart to deliver more blood to the muscles with each pulse of the heart.

In addition to collateral circulation, the body's supply of red blood cells is increased. There is thus more hemoglobin in the blood and the blood has a greater "oxygen-grabbing" capability. The result is that a significantly greater amount of oxygen can be carried per quart of blood.

Also, cardiac output, the amount of blood that the heart puts out with each beat, increases because of roving. The heart can thus do more work with each beat. Since the heart can do more work with the same number of beats, it can do the same work with fewer beats. Therefore, the heart rate drops for the rover. While the average American has a resting pulse rate in the neighborhood of 75, the rover's resting pulse may be as low as 45. This mean that the rover with a pulse rate of 45 saves about fifteen million heartbeats per year.

Another effect is an increased elasticity of the body's arteries. To transport blood effectively under differing need situations, the body's arteries must be able to contract their inside diameters on demand. In this country our arteries harden and become less elastic as we age, making such contraction more and more difficult. Roving has the effect of reversing this trend and causing the arteries to become more elastic rather than less and therefore easier to contract.

The above effects and many others, such as increased muscular flexibility and strength, are generated by the 2100 Exercise Program. As a result the body builds a strong capability to do work and to take sudden stress. Fatigue at any job, whether mental or physical, is slower to arrive. Likewise, sudden bodily stresses such as illness or accident are attended by less bodily damage and shorter recovery times. Not only does the body become more resistant to fatigue and stress, it also becomes more resistant to physical pain. A healthier body thus brings many capabilities to you that you could not ordinarily obtain. To sum up, the Program:

1. Develops new circulation;
2. Increases cardiac output;
3. Enables quicker recovery from illness and accident;
4. Decreases resting pulse rate;
5. Makes arteries more elastic;
6. Increases the blood's oxygen-grabbing power;
7. Enables the body to do more work with less effort;
8. Gives the body more resistance to injury and illness;
9. Makes the body more resistant to pain.

2100 PROGRAM ADVICE ON ROVING

Measuring Off Your Distance

Since roving revolves around a fixed distance that you select, you need to have some rough means of measuring distance. Your means of measurement do not have to be terribly accurate. If you drive and use your car's odometer to measure a few courses you wish to rove over and "guesstimate" on any other courses you wish to try, you will be doing fine. Some rovers like to get a topographical map of their area from the Federal government and use them to estimate course lengths. Other rovers like to buy a pedometer with which they can walk off the distances over their selected courses. A pedometer can be bought in any sporting goods store for around 10 dollars. Still others like to pace off distances by walking their courses with a "practiced" three-foot stride.* You can measure distance any way you please, and your measurements can be relatively rough, so you should have no difficulty in determining an appropriate roving course or two (or more) for yourself.

Normal Aches and Pains

Many rovers experience minor pains in their first few weeks of roving. This is quite normal and is usually of no consequence. A common complaint in the over-thirty crowd is lower back pain, particularly after long, slow roves. Low back pains usually result from poor posture, and simply by consciously paying attention to your roving posture and everyday posture you can quickly solve this problem. It invariably disappears with time and conditioning.

Another source of difficulty for many rovers is soreness in the knee, ankle, and hip joints. This kind of soreness will also go away with conditioning, but a joint very often must be handled tenderly. If you are experiencing joint pains, slow down. If you are walking, walk more slowly. Don't run on a sore joint unless you are pretty sure you are not injuring it. You may set yourself back a number of weeks if you do.

High-altitude Roving

Once you are really into the swing of roving you will want to do it wherever you go. You will particularly want to continue roving when you get into the mountains. But here is a word of caution: Your capabilities at sea level decrease rapidly as you gain altitude, and you cannot try to do as much at high altitudes as you are used to doing down at sea level. Allow for the altitude and scale yourself down accordingly. This is especially true for those who are just starting

---

* If your stride is close to three feet, it should take you close to 440 paces to complete a circuit of most high schools tracks. (Most high school tracks are quarter-mile tracks—440 yards.)

their 2100 Exercise Program and who have not yet fully reconditioned themselves and their hearts. It is a great deal easier to fibrillate the heart at higher-than-normal altitudes than it is at normal altitudes. So be careful, unless you feel confident that you are already fully reconditioned.

Footstrike

There are often questions about "footstrike"—that is, how the foot should meet the ground while running. The most common footstrike—and the least tiring for most runners—is the "heel-toe." In the heel-toe, the runner lands first on his heel, then rocks to his toe, and finishes the stride pushing off with his toe. Another footstrike is the "ball-of-the-foot" method in which the runner lands on and pushes off from the ball of the foot on every stride. This method can be very tiring to the calves and backs of the legs, but some runners prefer it. The third common footstrike method is flatfoot, in which the entire foot strikes the ground simultaneously. Flatfoot can be done in a soft and fluid manner and can be a very gentle stride.

The best advice on footstrike is to do whatever feels best to you. Knowing the three common footstrike methods may give you some ideas, but the best thing is to do what feels good and natural.

Posture

Since many of us have not run much since we were children, there are a number of awkward posture habits that tend to show up when we run. Although they will generally iron themselves out after you have been roving for a while (particularly for long-distance rovers), it is still worthwhile to consider them now. There are three primary things that control your posture when you run: Your head position, your arm position, and your leg action.

Head Position: Your head should be erect. By looking out and around you when you run, your head, spine, and hips tend to stay on a more or less vertical line. This sort of vertical posture is easy and natural and should not be confused with the military brace of head and shoulders back and chest out. The military brace is unnatural and tiring. Rather than the ramrod military posture, imagine that you are a puppet on a string that runs down through the top of your head and attaches to the centroid of your crotch area. The string forms a vertical centerline through your body, but your shoulders, arms, and legs are free to hang or move in any way about this centerline.

Arm Position: Your arms need to be carried low, drawn up only slightly from a natural hanging at your sides. Resist the temptation to draw your fists up high like a boxer or a sprinter. Keeping your arms down will increase the gracefulness of your stride and will save you energy.

Leg Action: The orientation of the different parts of your legs as your feet land and rebound again from the earth can make running hard or easy for you. The smoothest and most graceful stride is attained when all your running parts— your hips, upper leg, lower leg, ankle, and the length of your foot—stay in an ideal plane of action, which remains always vertical and parallel to your direction of motion. Figures 7 and 8 show the ideal plane of action as well as one of the common errors of running that happens when the leg action gets out of plane.

Figure 7 shows the ideal case, in which the planes of action are parallel to each other, and parallel to the line of motion of the runner. Figure 8 illustrates the shin splint case. Shin splints, an ancient complaint of runners, is caused by torn or inflamed connective tissue along the shin bone. Such damaged tissue is often caused by out-of-vertical planes of action. The most common cause of out-of-vertical

The 2100 Exercise Program 191

Figure 7. Ideal Case

Both planes are vertical, parallel to each other, and parallel to the direction of motion.

Direction of Motion

Left and Right Planes of Action

Plane of action tilted from vertical.

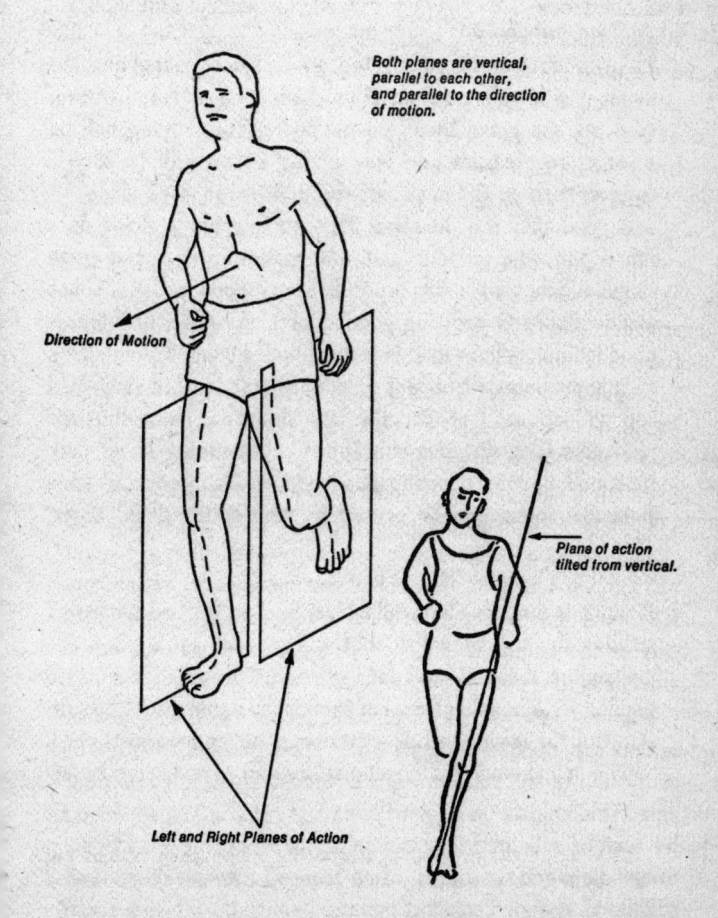

Figure 8. Shin Splint Case

planes of action, and therefore of shin splints, is shown in Figure 8. Here the runner is attempting to put one foot directly in front of the other as he runs instead of a little to the side. You can easily see that this throws his plane of action out of the vertical.

Surface and Shoes

The best surface for roving is grass or forest leaves and the worst is sidewalk cement. If you can rove on soft but firm surfaces like grass, by all means do so. Your roving will be a lot more pleasant and less jarring because of it. If you cannot, then do the next best thing: Rove in good shoes.

A good shoe is a shoe that fits your foot like a glove, does not slip around on your foot, and makes an even but cushioned contact with the ground. Many good calfskin shoes are available in sporting goods stores. A well-fitting tennis shoe is fine, so long as it is indeed well-fitting. Sometimes a simple crepe sole business shoe with soft leather sides and top will do just fine. But the best shoes are those that are made for long-distance running. Good running shoes may be found in most sporting goods stores. Hip joint and knee pain can sometimes be caused by improperly fitted shoes.

Forms of Exercise Other Than Roving *

Roving is a convenient, effective, and controlled means of gaining the sort of fitness that will protect you against degenerative diseases and increase your physical endurance capacity. Some other forms of exercise can sometimes be substituted for roving, while others can never be substituted.

The key to roving is that it enables you to raise your heart-

---

* Much of the material in this section comes from notions put forth by Roy Shephard in his book *Endurance Fitness* (University of Toronto, 1969).

beat to a certain rate (to between 140 and 180 beats per minute) and to keep it there for a sustained length of time, easily and in a controlled way.** Weekend sports such as skiing and ocean swimming have a high potential for the same effect, but in practice their effect is often slight. The individual often participates at far less than maximum capability, spending much time talking, changing, and watching other participants. Furthermore, the danger of overexertion in a short burst of activity is ever present for the over-thirty person.

Isometric exercises can never be substituted for roving. Such exercises not only do not increase the body's endurance fitness, but they even place a definite strain on the heart and the vascular system.

Competitive sports such as squash, tennis, handball, and basketball can be substituted for roving. Their endurance fitness potential is high, and they are to some extent controllable, in the sense that the pulse rate or the Heart Recovery Test can be periodically checked to determine the propriety of the exercise level. However, these sports require opponents, which can make them far less convenient than roving. In addition, with an opponent goes the feeling of competition and the element of risk of overexertion that can be dangerous for the person over thirty, at least in the beginning of endurance conditioning. This element of risk, however, disappears after a high level of endurance conditioning has been achieved.

Twisting, jumping, balancing, and agility exercises have little capability for endurance fitness but do have some capability for injury to at least the middle-aged participant. They cannot be used to replace roving. In the same way,

---

** Evidence shows that unless an elevated heart rate is sustained for at least 15 minutes, little endurance fitness will result.

weight lifting, while creating a body beautiful, does little to protect the body from degenerative diseases and does not provide endurance fitness. Weight lifting therefore cannot replace roving.

Both bicycle riding and the stationary bicycle can be substituted for roving. They both have the ability to raise the pulse rate and to maintain a raised pulse rate for controlled periods of time. Except for the fact that they require special equipment (which can be a drag on vacations, for example), they seem to have many of roving's advantages.

Regular swimming may be substituted for roving. Like roving, the heart rate can be raised and easily sustained at this raised level. Unlike roving, swimming often entails a considerable reliance on a fixed piece of property: a pool or a lake. Away from home, it may be difficult to find such necessary swimming facilities.

Roving and Problem Solving

All of us have problems to solve. Some of them may be business problems, some personal problems, or some may even be scientific problems. But whatever they are, they all need solving, and it turns out that roving is a very useful tool for solving them.

People who study problem solving tell us that we go about solving our problems in two stages. In the first stage we spend a lot of time worrying and thinking about what the problem is and what we might be able to do to solve it. Very often we find ourselves hopelessly deadlocked in this first stage. Our brain has worked and worked the problem but to no avail. Our thoughts are confused and muddled, and a solution to the problem seems hopeless. This is where the second stage of problem solving comes in.

The second stage is characterized by no attempt whatever to solve the problem. We give up. We forget about it for a while and go do something else. We turn our brain off and let our bodies function alone for a time. Then when we return later to the problem, perhaps the next day, the solution comes to us like a flash with little or no effort on our part.

Some people say that during the second stage our subconscious minds are solving the problem for us. Whether or not this is a correct way to view what is happening is debatable. The fact remains that this two-stage approach to problem solving works, and many great scientists have used it well to their own advantage. The key idea in the second stage is to drop the problem and to do something to refresh yourself. What better way to refresh yourself than to go out for a long rove. Roving can relieve your mind of your problems like nothing else can. A million years of human race history is packed into the rover's striding gait; it is the most natural form of physical refreshment you can take.

So when you have a knotty problem that simply will not yield to your attempts to analyze and solve it, drop it for a while and go roving. When you come back to the problem later, you may find that it is already solved.

Roving and Fear

Roving helps to dissolve fears. The fears that many people have of personal failure, physical abuse, or perhaps death will often yield under the pressure of continued roving. Somehow roving causes the thing that is feared to be less real and less important, and as a result the fear itself tends to melt away. People who are fearful of one thing or another can find great relief from long roves on a regular basis.

Roving and Age

People who live a long time have nearly always been active throughout their lives. Activity is absolutely necessary for an elderly person to keep the bones from growing brittle, the muscles from shrinking, and the organs from failing. For an old person physical activity buys him more life. Physical inactivity buys him a hurry-up funeral.

Physical activity for an old person usually cannot be football or even basketball. But it can be roving—lots of it. As much as he has time for. Dr. Paul Dudley White told of one of his patients, age 102, who had been walking all his life. Naturally, Dr. White's advice to the man was to keep on walking. He did keep on walking and lived to be 107. Our advice to the elderly is similar: Keep on roving.

Roving and Weight

Most overweight people try very hard to control their appetites and to be careful about what they eat. However, they are almost always unsuccessful over a long period of time. The reason that they are unsuccessful is not because they fail at self-control. Anyone in their situation, given their physical make-up, would fail just as consistently. The reason they are unsuccessful is that their appestat (the mechanism that controls their appetite) is set at too high a level. The appestat setting is by no means all in the mind. It is strongly influenced by diet (as we mentioned earlier) and by physical activity. Dr. Jean Mayer of Harvard in his book *Overweight* describes his observations of how the amount of food we eat is related to the amount of exercise we get. His observations are pictorially represented by Figure 9.

Figure 9 shows appestat level *versus* activity level. We have also shown in Figure 9 estimated hours of roving for each activity level. In this way we can get an idea of appestat level versus the amount of roving done.*

---

* Clearly this estimate is subject to wide variation, if for no other reason than that some people's one hour of roving will amount to more (or less) activity than other people's one hour of roving. The figure is intended for illustration rather than for numerical certitude.

The 2100 Exercise Program   197

Figure 9 shows us that the appestat level would be the highest if we were to rove 1, 2, or more hours every day. In fact, it gets increasingly higher as the number of hours of roving goes up. This makes sense: The more exercise we get, the more food we need to eat. But what is remarkable about Figure 9 is that the lowest appestat setting does not occur at zero hours of daily roving, but rather it is lowest at around a half hour of daily roving. This says that we tend to eat the least food when we exercise some (about a half hour) each day.

As it happens, overweight people tend to be in the cross-hatched region of Figure 9, where the physical activity level is low. The closer their activity level is to zero, the higher their appestat setting rises and the more overweight they tend to be. The striking conclusion we thus can draw is this: If you are overweight, you can do yourself a world of good by making sure your roves keep you going for somewhere in the neighborhood of a half hour each day. Furthermore, to prevent overweight it may be useful to insure that your roves extend over at least a half-hour period each day.

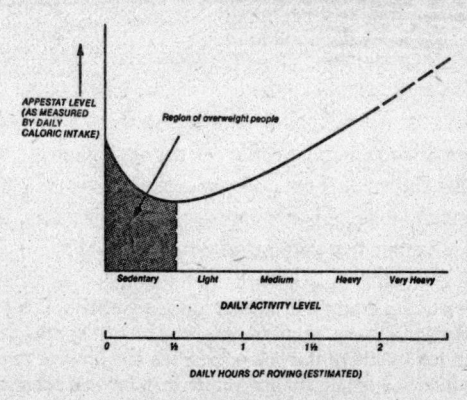

Figure 9. Appestat Level versus Activity Level

CHAPTER 9

Helpful Hints

From the last three chapters it is pretty clear that you stand to gain a lot from the 2100 Program. But all these chapters are just an academic exercise if you wind up dropping off the 2100 Program after you have been on it for a while. And as it happens there are plenty of pressures around to make it hard for you to stay with the program. You may as well know what some of these pressures are so that you can prepare yourself for them and not fall victim to them.

A Matter of Life Style

The 2100 Program is your way of getting what you need emotionally, physically, and nutritionally. Your 2100 Program is as important to your good health as is your night's rest. And just as your night's rest takes a certain amount of time from every 24-hour day, so does the 2100 Program take a certain amount of time from every day. It takes time, because only time spent doing your 2100 Program will give you the benefits you need. You cannot get 2100 results from 11 minutes a day, any more than you can get a good night's sleep in an hour and 15 minutes.

Unfortunately, you will undoubtedly find that our hectic modern life styles exert great pressure upon you to abandon your 2100 Program. People, schedules, and commitments will all try to take you away from it. All these things will be clamoring at you that there is no time in your life for your 2100 Program. But truly there is nothing more important to your personal health, and people, schedules, and commitments have no more right to take it away from you than they have to take away your night's rest.

To keep what is rightfully yours, you will have to make an important decision. You will have to decide how to put extra time into every day to attend to your new 2100 exercise and eating needs. This means that you will have to step to one side and let some things that were important to you slide on past you and out of your life.

How do you decide what to put out of your life? Only you can say. It is a terribly difficult thing for most people to do. Zen philosophers advise us that when we are cleaning up our lives to make ready for new things, we should not throw away the least important things, but rather we should throw away the most important things. Only in this way, they would say, can we gain complete mastery over our lives. This is awfully heavy medicine for the mind of Western man, and we only mention it to point out the magnitude of the problem some of us will have in making space for what we need. It is a big problem indeed.

Your Unwilling Family

If you are lucky, you and your whole family will take up the 2100 Program together. That is the most wonderful way in the world to get it started. You will be great reinforcement for each other to withstand the counterproductive pressures of your workaday lives and to withstand any early backsliding that may occur. You can plan your meals together, plan your rovings together, and in general enjoy a much heightened bond of family fellowship.

However, you may find yourself the only person in your family who is interested in the 2100 Program. If you are the person responsible for preparing the family meals, things will probably work out well. Your meal preparation job will simply be a little tougher. You will have to prepare two separate meals each mealtime: one for yourself and one for the rest of the family. However, cooking for one is very easy, and you'll soon learn to keep lots of things, such as vegetable stews and your favorite 2100 Program breads, handy for putting on the table. Above all, don't force the 2100 Food Program on your family just because you are in control of the kitchen. That is a good way to make enemies in the family, and, in addition, to sour them on the whole concept of the 2100 Program. Instead, set a good example for them and answer whatever questions they may have. Even encourage questions. Try hard, however, not to preach. This has exactly the same negative effect as force-feeding them 2100 Program food when they have not already accepted the 2100 ideas.

If you are not the person responsible for preparing the family food, things may get rather sticky. A wife may have her feelings utterly crushed by a husband who decides to switch to 2100 Program foods. Her cooking may be a very important part of her self-image, and the merest suggestion that she should change how she is cooking may be devastating. A husband in this situation must be very gentle and very wise indeed. If he is clever and lucky, his wife may agree to learn how to cook foods the 2100 way just for him.

On the other hand, you may simply wind up fixing your meals for yourself. You can expect some friction, particularly with the cook, whose kitchen you are now sharing. But things usually work out well, and you end up learning a lot about cooking and your own personal tastes.

Once again remember the cardinal rule: Do not preach to your family. Simply set a good example and answer any questions about the 2100 Program your family may have. You will probably find that after you have been on the program for awhile, half your family will have converted to it.

When Traveling

At home you can usually easily arrange your life in such a way as to accommodate the 2100 Eating and Exercise Programs. But when you are away from home, you may find yourself at the mercy of people and situations that do not easily lend themselves to the 2100 Program. On trips to see relatives or friends, you may find yourself having to choose between your 2100 Program and your relative's or your friend's food. When traveling on business your usual habit of using public restaurants for your meals will do violence to your 2100 Diet Program. Likewise the staples such as pancake mix and syrup that people take on camping trips also do violence to your 2100 Diet Program.

Any of these traveling situations can be adequately dealt with, if you plan and prepare for it in advance. The important thing to remember is that your ordinary sources of meals when traveling are usually not appropriate to the 2100 Program.

In most traveling situations, you will have ample opportunity to buy food from grocery stores during the trip. From the grocer you can obtain fruits, fruit juices, vegetables, allowable breads and crackers, and any kind of nonfat dairy product. These are all great for snacks and may be taken in the car in an ice chest and to a lesser extent on the plane or train. For elaborate, hot 2100 Program meals, you will have to plan ahead very carefully indeed. No 2100 Program restaurants exist at this time, so you will have to bring ingredients or utensils with you or find them as you go. Motels that come equipped with kitchenettes (there are some still in existence) may be of some help, if you are using motels for your sleeping quarters while you travel.

Roving is likewise not always as convenient on a trip as it is when you are home. However, there is usually plenty of roving that you can do on a trip if you simply stop and take time to do it. If you are traveling a lot on business, plan your business meetings to take place several hours after you arrive at your destination. Spend those several hours on long walks getting acquainted with the area. You will probably greatly improve your business effectiveness. On vacation trips by car, plan your travel legs so that you will have ample time for roving at the end of each day, wherever you may stop.

The Restaurant Situation

For some people, restaurant dining is a way of life that is not easily changed. People who live in an apartment containing no cooking or refrigeration facilities, for example, are literally forced to take their meals in a restaurant. If you are in this boat, you may as well know that there are no restaurants whose meals normally conform to the 2100 Program requirements, simple as these requirements are. The only way that you will be able to continue eating in restaurants and at the same time stay on the 2100 Diet Program is to induce the management or the chef to prepare your meals a little differently than the meals would normally be prepared. It is sufficient in most restaurants, for example, to induce the chef to prepare certain standard dishes (for example rice dishes, vegetable stews, bean dishes, meat loaves, spaghetti, and so forth) without any of the gremlin ingredients mentioned earlier: fat, sugar, salt, and cholesterol.* If you can get to know the chef well, you might even convince him to try his hand at one of the recipes listed earlier in this book. With a little luck the recipe he tries will become a specialty of the restaurant, and the chef and the management both will be appreciative of your contribution to their menu.

Most people, however, are not in this boat. They are not forced to eat in a restaurant on an everyday basis. Instead, they find themselves confronted with the restaurant situation only on an occasional basis.

Many social and business situations revolve around occasional dining at a nice restaurant. What should you do in these situations? To the extent that you can avoid these situations or direct them to something besides going out to eat, you should do so. However, it is unlikely that you can avoid or redirect all of them, and sometimes you are going to be stuck eating out in a restaurant. When this happens, there are several things that you can do.

One thing you can do is to jump off your 2100 Program for that one meal, and not worry about it. If you feel that you are the type of person that can hold fast to your 2100 convictions even while moving on and off the Program, and if your departures from the Program are only occasional, then by all means feel free to jump off now and then. Only you can decide about that. Many people, however, may be better off not to break their 2100 habits, even for one meal, because the constant pressure from society to depart from

---

* By no cholesterol, we mean less than 4 oz. of lean meat in your serving (actually only 4 oz. per day!) and no egg yolk, shellfish, organ meat (liver, heart, and the like), or animal skin.

the Program is so great anyway, that small departures soon become very big ones.

Most restaurants carry certain standard foods from which an assortment of allowable 2100 Program foods can be selected. Thus you can usually select main dishes with minimal amounts of fat and cholesterol, baked potatoes, tossed salads, juices, fruit, vegetables, nonfat milk, and decaffeinated coffee. However, it is important that the meats, potatoes, salads, and vegetables are prepared plain, without the normal sauces or toppings, which invariably are high-fat or sugar items. Likewise fried—especially deep-fried—items should be avoided.

People solve the restaurant situation in different ways. One woman solves her restaurant problems by eating at home in advance. When she goes to the restaurant, she orders the most inexpensive, lowest fat meal she can, then picks over it but doesn't really eat it.

Everyone develops his own way of handling the restaurant situation. When you develop yours, if you think others might be able to use it, drop us a line and tell us about it.

Eating at the Home of a Friend or Relative

Like the restaurant situation, your occasional dinners with friends or relatives can cause you to temporarily drop from the 2100 Diet Program. Do not worry about occasional deviations from the diet while eating at someone else's home. If your friends are sensitive to your interest in the 2100 Program, you may find them bending over backward to prepare meals that fit the program. But even if they are not, you can be somewhat choosy about what you eat and how much you eat, while violating no codes of social behavior.

Your Sometimes Sympathetic Co-workers

Your co-workers can be a help or a hindrance to you and your efforts to establish your 2100 Program. If they view your program as a "health nut" scheme, they may cause you some embarrassment over it. In the extreme, if they are sufficiently hostile, you may even be forced to abandon your program or face losing a functional relationship with your co-workers.

On the other hand your co-workers can really be a big help. They may become interested in the 2100 Program themselves, help you buy food for lunches, go out roving with you, and talk over your progress with you. Needless to say this situation is healthier and more productive for you than the former situation. Here are some hints to help you establish a good relationship with your co-workers rather than a bad one:

1. Do not preach.
2. Answer any questions you may get.
3. Buy a co-worker a copy of this book if he appears genuinely interested.
4. If your co-worker has a degenerative disease problem, explain how the 2100 Program can help him regain good health.
5. Overweight people are sometimes your best allies because they are almost always very diet-conscious and on the lookout for something that will help them. The 2100 Program will help them.

A 2100 Group in Your Area

You have to have a lot of strength to stay with the 2100 Program, because in our society following the program amounts to going against the grain of our entire system. Bucking the system is not easy. But it can be done, and it can be done single-handedly by anyone who really puts his mind to it.

To make things a lot easier and a lot more fun for yourself, however, you might think about getting a group of 2100 Programmers in your area together for your common good. There is no question that the more people in your environment who are into the program, the easier and more exciting it is for you. So if you want to get a group going, give it a try.

Starting Slowly on the 2100 Diet Program—Measuring Your Progress

Not everyone can embrace and adopt perfect 2100 Program eating habits in one fell swoop. Nor is it necessary to adhere 100 percent to the program from the beginning (or ever, for that matter). What is important is that the 2100 Diet Program eventually becomes your established way of eating for a large percentage of the time.

If you are a person who must adopt the 2100 Program on a gradual basis, then by all means do it gradually and do it in any way that is most convenient and appropriate for you. We are not going to recommend a fixed schedule by which you should make the transition to 2100 Program foods. That is pretty much up to you to decide. We are, however, going to recommend a method by which you may measure the progress you are making toward attaining your goal.

You can measure your progress by using the Diet Score Sheet shown in Figure 11. By filling in the blanks on this score sheet, you are able to keep a daily record of your diet score for an entire year. To determine the extent and the benefit of your progress, you need to look at your monthly scores. Your monthly scores can vary anywhere between zero and 248 points. If your monthly score is more than 50, it is likely that your diet program is effecting measurable health benefits in your body. Above 125, health benefits are large and grow larger at an accelerated rate. A score of more than 200 may be viewed as a score of maximum health benefit.* Figure 10 is an example of the monthly progress of a hypothetical individual using the scoring method of Figure 11. You may overlay your own monthly scores on the chart of Figure 10 to see how you are doing. Do not feel that the hypothetical individual whose progress is shown in the figure is to be held up as a goal which you should strive to equal or excel. You must set your own progress pace. The hypothetical individual is shown only as an example, not as a standard to meet.

* It should be noted that the only true measure of health benefit comes from decreasing fat, salt, sugar, and cholesterol in the diet. The scoring procedure outlined can only approximate this. While it seems to be good on the average, it is clearly possible to develop a fairly high score, while not sufficiently reducing fat, salt, sugar and cholesterol. For instance, a person eating small "perfect" meals might give himself a score of 7 each day, but if he subsequently gorges himself on snacks, ingesting many gremlin foods in the process, this score of 7 will be far too high for his real behavior.

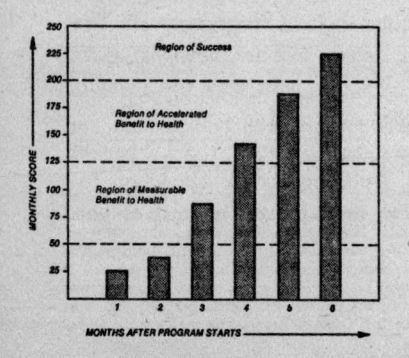

Figure 10.
Example of Progress in *2100 Program* as Measured by Monthly Scores for Six Months

Helpful Hints **209**

DIET SCORE* SHEET

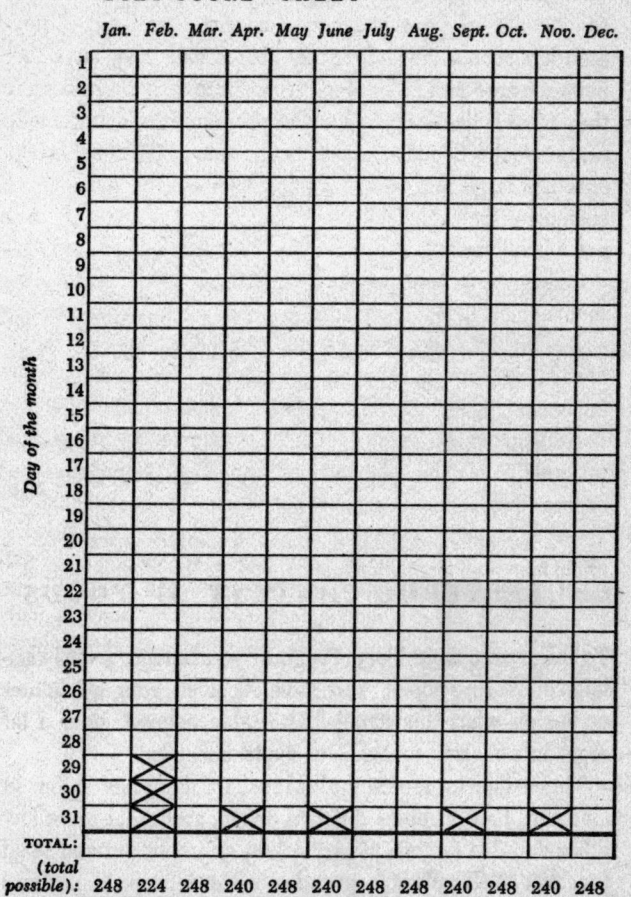

	Jan.	Feb.	Mar.	Apr.	May	June	July	Aug.	Sept.	Oct.	Nov.	Dec.
1												
2												
3												
4												
5												
6												
7												
8												
9												
10												
11												
12												
13												
14												
15												
16												
17												
18												
19												
20												
21												
22												
23												
24												
25												
26												
27												
28												
29		✕										
30		✕										
31		✕		✕		✕			✕		✕	
TOTAL:												
(total possible):	248	224	248	240	248	240	248	248	240	248	240	248

Day of the month

Figure 11. DIET SCORE SHEET FOR A YEAR.

* This score sheet has a space for every day of the year. At the end of each day, enter a daily score into the appropriate day. The daily score is figured on which meals were perfect (meaning 100 percent acceptable, or nearly so, according to the 2100 Program's five commandments for healthful eating). The daily score starts at zero. It grows, depending on which meals are perfect. If breakfast was perfect, add 2. If lunch was perfect, add 2 more. If dinner was perfect, add 3 more. If the snacks during the day were also perfect, add 1 as a bonus. Total possible score in a day is 8 (perfect score at all meals and snacks: $2 + 2 + 3 + 1$).

Appendix

CHOLESTEROL CONTENT OF FOODS

To follow the 2100 Food Program you have to avoid cholesterol-bearing foods. You have received your guidelines earlier on what this entails. The table below* gives a lot more information on what to avoid and why.

These figures are not absolute. Laboratories differ in methods, food samples differ in origin, and there are many other variable factors. Nevertheless, an important and valid function of this chart is to indicate the relative cholesterol values of different types of foods. For example, foods of animal origin always contain cholesterol, whereas foods derived from plants contain no cholesterol. The fact that meat or fish is lean does not necessarily indicate that it is low in cholesterol.

* This table is from *Low Cholesterol Diet Manual* prepared by the Department of Internal Medicine at the University of Iowa.

Approximate Amounts of Cholesterol in Milligrams Per 100 Gram (3½ Oz.) Portions of Foods

(Foods that should be excluded from this diet because of either their high cholesterol or high-fat content are listed in *italics*.)

BEEF	
Rump roast	58
Round steak	68
Chuck roast	55
VEAL	71
PORK	
Chops	55
Tenderloin	57
Ham	42
LAMB	
Chops	66
MUTTON	77
TURKEY—light	61
dark	96
CHICKEN—light	54
dark	76
Kidney	300
Liver, beef	320
Brains, calf	1810
Sweetbreads	280
Beef tallow	56
Lard	65

DAIRY PRODUCTS

MILK:	
Whole	14
Fortified skim (1% butterfat)	5
Skim	<1
Buttermilk	6
Butter	249
Cream—thick	140
Cream—thin	40
Egg yolk	1370
(1 egg yolk)	240

CHEESES:	
Limburger	92
Roquefort	73
Cream	140
American Process	87
Cheddar	98
Bleu	157
Mozzarella (part skim)	61
Swiss	91
Gouda	33
Hoop cheese	1
Parmesan	74
American	92

FISH	
Trout	57
Tuna	51

Salmon	55	SHELLFISH	
Halibut	33	*Shrimp*	161
Haddock	64	*Crab*	99
Codfish	46	*Lobster*	83
Mackerel	80	*Oysters*	161
Herring	75	*Scallops*	166
Perch	63	*Clams*	118
Pike	71		

Amounts of Cholesterol in Milligrams Per Serving of Food

1 Cup fortified skim milk (less than 1% buttermilk fat)	12	*1 Teaspoon butter*	10
		1 Tablespoon mayonnaise	15
1 Cup fortified skim milk (less than 0.5% butterfat)	6	*1 Tablespoon thick cream*	18
1 Cup skim milk	1	*Margarine, vegetable*	0
½ Cup sherbert	3	*Peanut butter*	0
1 Cup whole milk	35	Fruits	0
½ Cup ice cream	30	Vegetables	0
½ Cup ice milk	17	Egg whites	0
1 Egg yolk	240	Cereals	0
		Vegetable oils	0

COMPOSITION OF FOODS

The 2100 Food Program introduces ways of eating that will be unfamiliar to most readers. To those readers who have been conscious of the nutrient value of the foods they eat, the 2100 Program may be puzzling. For example, many people have been taught to regard liver as an indispensable part of their diet, because liver is high in certain nutrients, particularly iron. Since liver, because of its high cholesterol content, is excluded from the 2100 Program, one might naturally wonder where one's normal supply of iron would come from if liver is not to be eaten. The answer is that iron can be gotten from many, many acceptable foods, and this fact can be easily determined if one has access to a handbook which shows the composition of foods.

Undoubtedly the best handbook in existence on the subject is *Composition of Foods* by B. K. Watt and A. L. Merrill. Everyone interested in his health should have a copy of this classic 190-page handbook. It gives the vitamin, mineral, caloric, fat, protein, and carbohydrate content of literally thousands of common kitchen foods, in an easy-to-use format. It can be purchased from the Department of Agriculture or by sending $5.00 to Composition of Foods, P.O. Box 17873, Tucson, Arizona 85731.

The table reproduced on pages 232–235 is taken from Watt and Merrill's handbook. It shows the composition of the first five foods in the list of acceptable foods. Notice that iron can be found in significant quantities in every one of these foods, particularly in lima beans. (The iron content of mature lima beans actually exceeds that of beef liver.)

The table also exposes some interesting facts on the fat content of meat. Most of us have been used to thinking of meat as an important source of protein. But from the table, we can see that a favorite kind of steak (choice T-bone steak) is really mostly fat rather than protein. Although 55 percent of the T-bone steak is considered to be the "lean" part of the steak, over half of this lean is actually fat that is marbled through the piece of meat. And of course the "fat" part of the steak is almost 100 percent fat. Thus the T-bone steak turns out to be 71.7 percent fat and only 28.3 percent protein. Furthermore, the T-bone steak is not particularly high in fat as meat goes. Other kinds of steak (porterhouse, sirloin, chuck, etc.) and other forms of beef are also high in fat. It is also interesting to note that a pound of T-bone steak has only slightly more than *half* as much protein as a pound of pinto beans, red beans, white beans, etc. This fact is very surprising to most people, who view meat as the only important source of protein. It is not the only important source of protein. Considering the large quantities of fat and cholesterol that ordinarily accompany it, it is a *poor* source of protein.

Thus the sort of information that the table provides is very enlightening. Such information can settle many questions the reader may have concerning what nutrients the various foods have, and it will also illustrate the power of the 2100 Food Program to supply the basic nutrients that are needed for health. We reemphasize that the table is incomplete. It shows only the first few foods in the list of acceptable foods. Complete information can be found in *Composition of Foods*, mentioned on the previous page.

SIMPLIFIED USE AND AVOID LIST

	Use	*Avoid*
MEAT * FISH * BEANS NUTS EGGS	Chicken, turkey, veal, fish, beef (lean), lean hamburgers Trim all visible fat before cooking. Bake, broil, roast or stew. Dried beans and peas Eggs—whites only	Lamb, pork, ham, duck, (limit) Shellfish, shrimps Marbled and fatty meats—spareribs, mutton, frankfurters, sausages, fatty hamburgers, bacon, luncheon meats Organ meats—liver, kidney, heart, sweetbreads Eggs—no yolks Nuts—none
VEGETABLES FRUITS	All fruits and vegetables raw, baked, boiled Limit dried fruit (raisins 1 oz. per day, prunes and other fruits 2 oz. per day)	Olives and avocados

* Limit intake of meat and fish to a total of 3 to 4 ounces daily.

BREADS CEREALS	Sourdough bread, any other bread without shortening or sugar Rice, pasta, noodles (except egg noodles) Spaghetti Any cold cereal without shortening or sugar, as shredded wheat Any hot cereal without shortening or sugar, as oatmeal	Any baked goods with shortening and/or sugar, such as cakes, crackers, donuts, sweet rolls, commercial mixes with dried eggs and whole milk
MILK PRODUCTS	Milk, skim (nonfat) Cheese made from skim (nonfat) milk, as farmer's, baker's, or hoop cheese	Chocolate milk, canned whole milk, powdered whole milk, creams, yogurt with butterfat and sugar, nondairy cream substitutes Cheeses—all cheeses except skim milk cheeses
FATS & OILS	None	Butter, lard, meat fat, margarine, all oils
DESSERTS BEVERAGES SNACKS CONDIMENTS	Fresh fruit * and canned fruit * (not in syrup) Crackers, bread or rolls without shortening or sugar Decaffeinated beverages Herb teas	Puddings, ice cream, sherbets Canned fruit in syrup Gelatin desserts Fried foods, as potato chips All bakery items containing shortening and sugar Sugared drinks Candy Salt (do not add to food)

* At the start of your 2100 Program limit fruit to 4 pieces per day and limit fruit juices to 4 oz. per day (or limit fruit and fruit juices, taken together, to 15–20 percent of total calories). The simple sugar fructose is a major constituent of fruits. Fructose can be a powerful raiser of blood fat levels; for this reason the amount of fruit and fruit juices must be limited at the start. Once your blood fat levels have been reduced to low 2100 Program levels (60 mg. % of triglycerides and 500 mg. % for total lipids), this fruit limitation will probably no longer be necessary.

EXTENDED LIST OF ACCEPTABLE FOODS

This list is not meant to be all-inclusive. Just because something is not on the list does not mean that it is unacceptable. The list is simply intended to be a resource list to expand your ideas of what you can eat.

Many of the foods listed can be obtained in fresh, frozen, canned, or dry form. Avoid these foods when packaged with sugar, fats, or special additives. Since the fruit-drying process ordinarily causes some simple sugar to crystallize on the fruit, dried fruits should be limited to two ounces per day.

- Apples
- Apple juice
- Apple sauce
- Apricots
- Asparagus
- Bananas
- Barley (pearled)
- Beans (white, red, pinto, calico, red Mexican, black, brown, Bayo, lima)
- Bean sprouts
- Beef (lean steak, roasts, hamburger)
- Beets
- Blackberries
- Blueberries
- Breads
- Breakfast foods:
  - Nabisco Shredded Wheat
  - Roman Meal
  - Post Grapenuts
  - Cream of Wheat (Regular)
  - Quaker Oats (Old Fashioned, Quick, Rolled)
  - Quaker Grits
  - Cornmeal
  - Wheat Hearts
  - Wheat Nuts
  - Wheatena
  - Cracked wheat
- Broccoli
- Brussel sprouts
- Buckwheat flour
- Cabbage (red or green)
- Cantaloupe
- Carrots
- Cauliflower
- Celery
- Chard
- Cheeses:
  - Cottage cheese (made from skim milk)
  - Farmer's cheese
  - Hoop cheese

Appendix 217

Cherries
Chicken (without skin)
Chickpeas or garbanzos
Collards
Corn
Cornbread
Corn grits
Cow peas
Crackers (no saltines)
Cranberries
Cucumbers
Currants
Eggplant
Endive or escarole
Farina
Fish:
  Bluefish, cod, flounder,
  haddock, halibut, herring,
  mackerel, salmon, trout,
  whitefish
Grapefruit
Grapefruit juice
Grapefruit-orange juice
Grapes
Grape juice
Guavas
Honeydew melon
Kale
Kohlrabi
Lemons
Lemon juice
Lentils
Lettuce
Limes
Loganberries

Macaroni (without eggs)
Mangos
Milk (skim, dried skim)
Mushrooms
Muskmelons
Mustard greens
Nectarines
Noodles (without eggs)
Oat cereal
Oatmeal or rolled oats or
  steel-cut oats
Okra
Onions
Oranges
Papayas
Parsley
Parsnips
Peaches
Peas
Peppers (green or red bell
  peppers)
Persimmons
Pimientos
Pineapple
Pineapple juice
Plums
Potatoes
Prunes
Prune juice
Pumpkin
Radishes
Raisins
Raspberries
Rhubarb
Rice (brown, wild)

Appendix

- Rutabagas
- Unsalted rye wafers
- Sauerkraut
- Soups (without sugar, oil, or additives)
- Soybeans
- Spaghetti
- Spinach
- Squash (all varieties)
- Strawberries
- Sweet potatoes
- Tangerines
- Tomatoes
- Tomato juice
- Tortillas (corn)
- Turkey
- Turnips
- Turnip greens
- Veal (lean)
- Vinegar
- Watermelon
- Wheat flours (whole, unbleached)

Source Notes

1. U.S. Bureau of the Census, *U.S. Vital Statistics* (for years 1910 through 1967).
2. International Society of Cardiology, *Bulletin of the International Society of Cardiology*, 1: 1–10 (1969).
3. Enos, et al., "Pathogenesis of Coronary Disease in American Soldiers Killed in Korea," *JAMA*, July 16, 1955.
4. McNamara, J. J., et al., "Coronary Artery Disease in Vietnam Casualties," *JAMA*, May 17, 1971.
5. Moss, A. J., "Ballisticardiographic Evaluation of the Cardiovascular Aging Process," *Circulation*, 23: 435–451, March 1961.
6. Kuller, L., et al., "Epidemiological Study of Sudden and Unexpected Deaths Due to Atherosclerotic Heart Disease," *Circulation*, 34, December 1966.
7. Keys, A., et al., "Coronary Heart Disease Among Minnesota Business and Professional Men Followed Fifteen Years," *Circulation*, 27, September 1963.
8. Kannel, W. B., et al., *Am. J. Pub. Health*, 55: 1355 (1965).
9. Keys, A., "Coronary Heart Disease in Seven Countries," *Circulation*, 41, Supplement 1 (1970).

10. Rosenman, R. H., *et al.*, "Comparative Predicted Value of Three Serum Typed Entries in a Prospective Study of CHD," *Circulation*, 35, Supplement 2 (1967).
11. Hannah, J. B., "Civilization, Race, and Coronary Atheroma with Particular Reference to its Severity in Africans," *Central African J. Med.*, 4: 1–5 (1958).
12. Walker, A. P., *et al.*, "Glucose and Fat Tolerances in Bantu Children," *Lancet*, p. 51, July 4, 1970.
13. Whyte, H. M., *Aust. Ann. Med.*, 7: 36–37 (1958).
14. Leaf, A., "Hard Labor, Low Cholesterol Linked to Unusual Longevity," *Medical Tribune*, June 1971.
15. Keys, A., *et al.*, "Lessons from Serum Cholesterol Studies in Japan, Hawaii, and Los Angeles," *Ann. Int. Med.*, 48: 83–94 (1958).
16. Taylor, C. B., *et al.*, "Atherosclerosis in Rhesus Monkeys," *Archives of Pathology*, 76: 404 (1963).
17. McGill, H. C., "Geographic Pathology of Atherosclerosis," *Lab. Invest.*, 18: 463 (1968).
18. Leren, P., "The Oslo Diet-Heart Study," *Circulation*, 62: 935 (1970).
19. Report to Medical Research Council, "Controlled Trial of Soybean Oil," *Lancet*, 693, September 28, 1968.
20. Dayton, S., *et al.*, "Controlled Trial of Diet High in Unsaturated Fat," *Circulation*, Supplement 2, article number 1 (1969).
21. Gresham, *et al.*, "Thrombogenesis in Rats," *Fed. Proc.*, 22: 1371, pt. 1 (1963).
22. Getz, G. S., *et al.*, "Lipids in Rhesus Monkeys," *Circulation*, Supplement 2, 35: 11–13 (1967).
23. Joyner, C. R., *et al.*, "Effect of Anxiety on Atherosclerosis in Cockerels," *Circulation Research*, 9: 69 (1961).
24. Vahouny, G. V., *et al.*, "Effect of Cold on Atherosclerosis," *Fed. Proc.*, Part I, 367, March 1961.
25. Hinkle, L. E., "Heart Disease Among Lower Executives," *JAMA*, 204: 41 (1968).
26. Barnes, B. O., *et al.*, "Arteriosclerosis in 10,000 Autopsies," *Fed. Proc.*, 19: 19 (1960).
27. Armstrong, M. C., *et al.*, "Regression of Coronary Athero-

matosis in Rhesus Monkeys," *Circulation Research 27:* 59 (1970).

28. Tucker, C., et al., "Regression of Cholesterol-induced Atherosclerotic Lesions in Rhesus," *Circulation, Supplement 2, 63:* 48 (1971).

29. Reaven, G. M., et al., "Study of the Relationship Between Plasma Insulin Concentrations and Efficiency of Glucose Uptake in Normal and Mildly Diabetic Subjects," *Diabetes, 19:* 571–578 (1970).

30. Reaven, G. M., et al., "Steady State Plasma Insulin Response to Continuous Glucose Infusion in Normal and Diabetic Subjects," *Diabetes, 18:* 273–279 (1969).

31. Reaven, G. M., et al., "Is There a Delay in the Plasma Insulin Response of Patients with Chemical Diabetes Mellitus," *Diabetes, 20:* 416–423 (1971).

32. Buber, V., "Improvement of Oral Glucose Tolerance by Acute Drug Induced Lowering of Plasma Free Fatty Acids," *Schweiz. Med. Wschr., 98:* 711–712 (1968).

33. Groen, et al., "Effect of Interchanging Bread and Sucrose as Main Source of Carbohydrate on Cholesterol Level," *American J. Clin. Nutr., 19:* 46–58 (1966).

34. Cohen, A. M., et al., "Effect of Interchanging Bread and Sugar as Main Source of Carbohydrate on Glucose Tolerance," *Amer. J. Clin. Nutr., 19:* 59–62 (1966).

35. Campbell, G. D., "Diabetes in Asians and Africans in and Around Durham," *South African Med. J., 37:* 1195 (1963).

36. Antones, A., et al., "The Influence of Diet on Serum Triglycerides," *Lancet, 1:* 3 (1961).

37. "University Group Diabetes Program," *Diabetes, Supplement 2, 19* (1970).

38. "Pioneer in Study of Insulin Dies at 88," *JAMA, 218:* 25 (1971).

39. "Diabetes Study Head Assails Critics," *Medical Tribune,* November 1970.

40. White, P. D., et al., "Coronary Heart Disease in Former Football Players," *JAMA, 267:* 711 (1958).

41. Taylor, H. L., et al., "Death Rates Among Physically Active and Sedentary Employees of the Railroad Industry," *Amer. J. Pub. Health, 52:* 1697 (1962).

42. Frank, C. W., et al., "Physical Inactivity as a Lethal Factor in Myocardial Infarction Among Men," *Circulation*, 34: 1022 (1966).
43. Kidera, "Exercise Aids in Converting ECG to Normal," (Medical News), *JAMA*, 204: 31 (1968).
44. Laurie, W., "Prevention of Myocardial Infarction," *Med. J. Australia*, 1: 361–363 (1971).
45. Bloor, *Lab. Invest.*, 22: 160 (1970).
46. Eckstein, R. W., "Effect of Exercise and Coronary Artery Narrowing on Coronary Collateral Circulation," *Circulation Research*, 5: 230 (1957).
47. Tepperman, J., et al., "Effects of Exercise and Anemia on Coronary Arteries of Small Animals as Revealed by the Corrosion-Cast Technique," *Circulation Research*, 9: 576 (1961).
48. Jokl, E., "Exercise and Cardiac Death," *JAMA*, 218: 1707 (1971).
49. Menon, I. S., et al., "Effect of Strenuous and Graded Exercise on Fibrinolytic Activity," *Lancet*, 700, April 1, 1967.
50. Angelino, P. F., et al., "Physical Activity and Fibrinolysis," *Minerva Med.*, 55: 2111, July 4, 1964. (Translation in JAMA: 190)
51. Ogston, D., et al., "Changes in Fibrinolytic Activity Produced by Physical Activity," *Lancet*, 2: 730, September 30, 1961.
52. Winther, O., "Exercise and Fibrinolysis," *Lancet*, 1195, November 26, 1966.
53. Rosing, D. R., "Blood Fibrinolytic Activity in Man," *Circulation Research*, 27: 171–184, August 1970.
54. Carlstrom, S., et al., "Plasma Free Fatty Acids in Diabetics During Exercise," *Lancet*, 331: February 8, 1964.
55. "Controlled Exercise Cuts Diabetic Symptoms," *Medical Tribune*, July 14, 1971.
56. Luyken, R., et al., "Nutrition Studies in New Guinea," *Amer. J. Clinical Nutrition*, 14: 13–27 (1964).
57. Chance, G. W., et al., "Serum Lipids in Diabetic Children," *Lancet*, pp. 1126–1128, June 7, 1969.
58. Bagdade, J. D., "Diabetic Lipemia," *New England J. Med.*, 276: 427–433 (1967).

59. "Present Knowledge of Nutrition in Diabetes," *Nutrition Reviews, 24:* 254–260 (1966).
60. Yudkin, J., "Dietary Fat and Dietary Sugar in Relation to Ischemic Heart Disease and Diabetes," *Lancet,* pp. 4–5, July 4, 1954.
61. Wada, S., et al., *Diabetes 13:* 485 (1964).
62. Conner, W. E., *Diabetes 12:* 127 (1963).
63. Hsueh-Li, C., et al., *Chinese Med. J. 84:* 451 (1965).
64. *Statistical Bulletin 45:* 7 (August 1964).
65. *Statistical Bulletin 46:* 1 (August 1965).
66. *Medical World News 6:* 146 (1965).
67. Wolf and Priess, "Fat Free Diet in Diabetes Mellitus," *Deutsche Med. Wehnschr. 81:* 514–515 (1956).
68. Marble, A., *Med. World News 6:* 146 (1965).
69. Gerson, T., et al., *Biochem J. 81:* 584 (1961).
70. Wissler, R. W., et al., *Arch. Path 74:* 312 (1962).
71. Friedman, M., et al., *JAMA 193:* 882 (1965).
72. Bierenbaum, M., et al., *Circulation 42:* 943 (1970).
73. Rinzler, S. H., "Prevention of Heart Disease by Diet," *Bull. N. Y. Acad. Med. 44:* 936–949.
74. Turpeinen, O., et al., "Diet and Coronary Events," *J. American Diet. Association 52:* 209–213 (1968).
75. Morrison, L. M., "Diet in Coronary Atherosclerosis," *JAMA 173:* 884–888 (1960).
76. Hood, B., et al., "Long-Term Prognosis in Essential Hypercholesteremia," *Acta Med. Scand. 178:* 161–173 (1965).
77. Nelson, A. M., "Treatment of Atherosclerosis by Diet," *Northwest Med.,* pp. 643–649 (1956).
78. Hansen, P. F., et al., "Dietary Fats and Thrombosis," *Lancet,* pp. 1193–1194 (Dec. 1962).
79. Rose, G. A., et al., "Corn Oil in Treatment of Heart Disease," *Brit. Med. J.,* pp. 1531–1533, June 12, 1965.
80. Ball, K. P., et al., "Low Fat Diet in Myocardial Infarction," *Lancet,* pp. 501–504, Sept. 11, 1965.
81. Zukel, W. J., "Multiple Risk Factor Intervention Trial," An RFP (Number 73–11) from the Office of the Associate Director for Clinical Applications, National Heart and Lung Association, Department of Health, Education and Welfare, Bethesda, Maryland (1973).

82. "Coronary Drug Project," *JAMA 214*: 1303 (1970).
83. "Coronary Drug Project," *JAMA 220*: 996 (1972).
84. Karpovich, P. V., *Physiology of Muscular Activity*, W. B. Saunders Co., 1962, Chapter 13.
85. Medical News, "High Pressure Fails to Break Cerebral Arteries," *JAMA 210*: Dec. 8, 1969.
86. Shoenberger, et al., "Current Status of Hypertension Control," *JAMA 222*: 559–562, Oct. 30, 1972.
87. Beeson and McDermott, *Textbook of Medicine*, W. B. Saunders Co., 1971, pp. 1050–1062.
88. Evans, P. H., "Relation of Long Standing Blood Pressure Levels to Atherosclerosis," *Lancet*, p. 516, March 6, 1965.
89. Krupp, M. A., et al., *Physicians Handbook*, 16th Ed., Lange Medical Publications (1970), p. 54.
90. Perera, G. A., and Blood, D. W., "The Relationship of Sodium Chloride and Hypertension," *J. Clin. Invest. 26*: 1109 (1947).
91. Dole, V. P., et al., "Dietary Treatment of Hypertension," *J. Clin. Invest. 30*: 1189 (1951).
92. Blair-West, et al., "Sodium Homeostasis, Salt Appetite, and Hypertension," *Circulation Research 26 & 27; Supplement 2*: 258 (Oct. 1970).
93. Dahl, L., "Possible Role of Salt in Hypertension," *Essential Hypertension*, Springer-Verlag, 1963, p. 53.
94. Fries, E. D. and Sappington, R. F., "Long Term Effect of Probenecid on Diuretic-Induced Hypoglycemia," *JAMA 198*: 147 (1966).
95. Watts, R. W. E., et al., "Microscopic Studies on Muscle with Allopurinol," *Quart. J. Med. 40*: 1–14, 1971.
96. Dustan, H. P., et al., "Arterial Pressure Responses to Discontinuing Hypertensive Drugs," *Circulation 37*: 370–379 (March 1968).
97. *Information Please Almanac—1971*, Dan Golenpaul Associates, New York, p. 681.
98. Strehler, B. L., "Consequences of the Understanding of Aging," *Proceedings of the Life Span Conference*: April 13–17, 1970, Center for the Study of Democratic Institutions, Santa Barbara, California (1970).

99. Kurtzke, J. F., *Epidemiology of Cerebrovascular Disease*, Springer-Verlag, New York, 1969, p. 114.
100. Fries, E. D., "Chemotherapy of Hypertension," *JAMA 218*: 1009–1015.
101. National Center for Health Statistics, *Change in Mortality Trend in the U. S.*, Series 3, Number 1, Vital and Health Statistics Analytical Studies, HEW, Washington, D.C., March 1964.
102. Keys, A. (quotations from the article "Atherosclerosis"), *JAMA 5*: 290–294 (1957).
103. *Scientific American*, September 1971.
104. Yalow, R. S., and Berson, S. A., "Immunoassay of Endogenous Plasma Insulin in Man," *J. Clin. Invest. 39*: 1157–1175 (1960).
105. Barclay, W. R., "Tolbutamide: More Questions than Answers," *JAMA 215*: 108–109 (1971).
106. Mann, G. V., et al., *J. Atheroscler. Res. 4*: 289 (1964).
107. Mann, G. V., *et al.*, "Physical Fitness in Masai," *Lancet*, Dec. 25, 1965, pp. 1308–1310.
108. Garret, L., et al., *Fedn. Proc., Fedn. Am. Socs. Exp. Biol. 24*: Abstracts, 1965.
109. Hanson, J. and Nedde, W., "Physical Training for Hypertensive Males," *Circulation Research 26 & 27, Suppl. 1*: 49–53 (July 1970).
110. Wohl, M. G. and Goodhart, R. S., *Modern Nutrition in Health and Disease*, 4th Ed., Lea & Febiger, Philadelphia, 1968.
111. Watt, B. K., and Merrill, A. C., *Composition of Foods*, USDA Handbook No. 8, 1963.
112. Hardinge, M. C., and Crooks, H., *J. Amer. Dietet. Assoc. 34*: 1065 (1958).
113. Williams, R. J., *Nutrition in a Nutshell*, Doubleday, 1962.
114. Food and Nutrition Board, *Recommended Dietary Allowances*, 7th Ed., National Academy of Sciences, Washington, D. C., Publication 1694 (1968).
115. Wagner, A. F. and Folkers, K., *Vitamins and Coenzymes*, Interscience Publishers, 1964.
116. Winitz, M., *et al.*, "Evaluation of Chemical Diets," *Nature*, *205*: 741–743, February 20, 1965.

117. Beck, C. S. and Leighninger, D. S., "Scientific Basis for the Treatment of Coronary Disease," *JAMA* 159: 1264, November 26, 1955.
118. Mayer, J., *Overweight*, Engelwood Cliffs, N.J.: Prentice-Hall, Inc., 1968.
119. Mayer, J., *Medical Tribune* (quotation), January 19, 1970.
120. WHO, *World Health Statistical Annual—1968*, Geneva, 1971.
121. Public Health Service, *Smoking and Health*, PHS Publication No. 1103, 1964, p. 5.
122. Ibid., p. 26.
123. Ibid., p. 29.
124. Ibid., p. 30.
125. Public Health Service, *Health Consequences of Smoking, 1968 Supplement*, PHS Publication Number 1696, 1968.
126. Paul, O., et al., "Study of Coronary Heart Disease," *Circulation* 28: 20–31 (1963).
127. Jankelson, O. M., et al., "Effect of Coffee on Glucose Tolerance," *Lancet*, 527–529, March 11, 1967.
128. Bellet, S., et al., "Response of Free Fatty Acid to Coffee and Caffeine," *Metabolism* 17: 702–708 (1968).
129. Bellet, S., et al., "Effect of Caffeine on Ventricular Fibrillation Threshold," *Amer. Heart J.* 84: 215–227 (1972).
130. Kuhlmann, W., et al., "Mutagenic Action of Caffeine," *Cancer Research* 28: 2375–2389 (November 1968).
131. Himsworth, H. P., The Dietetic Factor Determining the Glucose Tolerance and Sensitivity to Insulin of Healthy Men. *Clin. Sci.* 2: 67–94, 1935.
132. Felber, J. P. and Vannotti, A., "Effects of Fat Infusion," *Medicina Experimentalis*, 10: 153–156 (1964).
133. Sweeney, J. S., "Dietary Factors That Influence Tolerance Tests," *Arch. Int. Med.*, 40: 818–830 (927).
134. Rabinowitch, I. M., "Effects of High Carbohydrate Diet on Diabetes," *Canadian Med. Assoc. J.*, Aug. 1935, pp. 136–144.

Index

Acapulco Brown Rice, 173
Age, roving and, 195–96
Alcoholism, 105
Allopurinol, 72
American Heart Association, 38
American Medical Association, 62
   Journal of, 78
Amino acids (proteins), 103
   carbohydrates and, 89, 90
   nutrition and, 94–98
Aneurysms ("blowouts"), 67
Animals, heart disease in, 29–30
Armstrong, M. L., 36
Arterial hypertension, 4, 6
   defined, 18–19
   See also Hypertension
Arteries
   atherosclerosis and, 31–35
   blood pressure and, 64–68
Arteriosclerosis, defined, 18
Arthritis, 72
Atherosclerosis, 4, 18–48
   arterial breakdown and, 31–35
   cholesterol and, 32–35, 142
   defined, 18–20
   diabetes and, 58–59
   heart disease and, 18, 20
   hypertension and, 69
   possible deaths due to, 4
   reversal of, 35–37
   study of, 21
Austria, heart disease in, 46
Autumn Bean Dressing, 161

Baltimore, heart disease in, 14
Banting, F. G., 49
Bantus
   diabetes among, 54
   heart disease among, 26–27
Beck, Claude, 79
Bellet, Samuel, 75

Beriberi, 99
Berson, S. A., 51
Bierenbaum, Marvin, 40
Blaiberg, Philip, 144
Blood pressure
   heart disease and, 23
   hypertension and, 64–68
   in U.S., 27
"Blowouts" (aneurysms), 67
Bolivia, life expectancy in, 16
Breading, 158
Breads, 147, 149–50, 215
Briny Deep Salmon Loaf, 168
Browning, 157–58
"Build and Blood Pressure Study"
   (Society of Actuaries), 65
Buttermilk Spring Dressing, 160
Buys, F. J., 83–84

Cabbage/Beet Borscht, 164
Caffeine, 75–76, 143–44
Carbohydrates
   nutrition and, 89–94
   sugar diabetes and, 55–58
Cereals, 147–49, 215
Cerebral hemorrhage, aneurysms
   and, 67
Cerebral infarction, 20
Cerebrovascular disease (stroke), 4
   aneurysms and, 67
   atherosclerosis and, 20
   possible death due to, 5, 6
Champion Crabbet, 180
Chicken, *see* Poultry
Chicken Fricassee with Vegetables
   and Dumplings, 170–71
Cholesterol
   atherosclerosis and, 32–35, 142
   content of foods, 210–12
   degenerative disease and, 142
   diet and, 146

Index

heart disease and, 22–30
-lowering drugs, 46–48
unsaturated fats and, 39–44
Cigarette smoking, degenerative diseases and, 73–74
Clofibrate, 47
Coffee, degenerative diseases and, 75–76, 143, 145
Competitive sports, 193
Composition of Foods (Watt and Merrill), 213, 214
Conjugated estrogens, 47
Conner, W. E., 53, 55
Constipation, 105
Cooking, tips for, 155–58
Cornfield, Jerome, 41
Coronary Drug Project (CDP), 47–48
Crackers, 150

Dahl, L. K., 70
Dairy foods, 150–51, 215
cholesterol content of, 211–212
nonfat, 146
Deaths, due to degenerative diseases, 6–8
Degenerative diseases
causes of, 73–76
deaths due to, 6–8
defined, 4–5
exercise and, 77
nutrition and, 141–44
See also Atherosclerosis; Cerebrovascular disease; Diabetes; Heart disease; Hypertension
Diabetes, 4, 6, 48–63
defined, 18
exercise and, 83–84, 178
fats and, 52–63
insulin and, 49–53
possible deaths due to, 140
Diarrhea, 105
Diets
fad, 122–27
importance of, 144–47
low-fat, 38, 55–59
low fat/low cholesterol, 25–26, 30, 36–37, 41–43
2100 food program and, 140–77
Diet Score Sheet, 207, 209
Diet Watchers, 124
Dinners, planning, 153–54
Dressings
Autumn Bean, 160

Buttermilk Spring, 160
Mock Sour Cream, 161
Dried foods, 152
Drugs
for diabetes, 60–63
for hypertension, 71–72
DT 4, 47

Ecuador, heart disease in, 27
Eggplant, breading of, 158
Emotional stress, 44–46
Enchiladas de Tijuana, 172–73
Endurance Fitness (Shepard), 192n
Entrees
Italian, 165–67
sea food, 168–69
from south of the border, 172–73
specialty, 170–72
Enzyme, 103
Ernst, Mensen, 179
Estrogens, 47
Exercise
diabetes and, 83–84, 178
heart disease and, 78–81, 178
hypertension and, 81–83
2100 Program of, 178–98

Fad diets, 122–27
Farmers' Onion-Cheese Pie, 172
Fats (and oils)
atherosclerosis and, 32–35
carbohydrates and, 90
degenerative diseases and, 141–42
diabetes and, 52–55, 58
diet and, 25–26, 30, 36–38, 41–43, 55–59, 145, 147
food composition of, 213–215
heart disease and, 23–30
skimming of, 157
unsaturated fats and, 39–44
Fatty acids, 114
caffeine and, 143
Fear, roving and, 195
Fibrillation, 10
Finland, heart disease in, 11
Fish, 146, 151, 214
breading, 158
cholesterol content of, 212
Food and Drug Administration (FDA), 62
Food industry, 116–22
Foods, *see* Nutrition

Index

Framingham (Mass.), Public Health Service study in, 23, 78
Franklin, Benjamin, 128
Fresh Frozen Pea Soup, 104
Friedman, Meyer, 40
Fruits, 146, 152, 214
Funk, Casimir, 98–99, 101, 104

Gangrene, 20
Garret, L., 82
Gazpacho (Spanish Salad Soup), 162–63
Gout, 4, 6
Greece, heart disease in, 11
Green Lentil Soup, 161–62
Groen, J. J., 56
Guinness Book of World Records, 179–80

Hanson, John, 82–83
Hayward, Wally, 180
Health, Education, and Welfare, U.S. Department of (HEW), 15
Health food stores, 129–31
Heart, the
  atherosclerosis and blood in, 78–80
  roving and, 186
Heart disease, 4, 8–15
  atherosclerosis and, 18, 20
  cigarette smoking and, 74
  coffee drinking and, 75–76
  emotional stress and, 44–46
  exercise and, 78–81, 178
  fats and cholesterol and, 24–30
  possible deaths due to, 5, 6, 136, 140
  study of, 21–24
  unsaturated fats and, 37–44
Heart Recovery Test, 183
"High Protein Diet," 126–27
Hinkle, L. E., 45
Holiday Salad, 160
Hood, B., 42, 43
Hormone, 102, 103
Hypertension, 64–72
  causes of, 68–71
  exercise and, 81–83
  high blood pressure and, 64–68
  treating, 71–72
Hypoglycemia, 49, 58, 94

Infarction, 9
Infective disease
  curing of, 4
  deaths due to, 6–8
Insulin
  blood sugar and, 56–58
  diabetes and, 49–53, 60–63
  low-fat diet and, 59
  simple sugars and, 94
Isometric exercises, 193
Italian entrees, 165–67
Italy, heart disease in, 11

Jankelson, Oscar, 75
Japan
  heart disease in, 11
  hypertension in, 70, 143
  low-fat diet in, 27–28
Joslin Clinic (Boston), 62
Journal of the American Medical Association, 78
Juices, 151

Keys, Ancel, 22–23, 28
Kidera (researcher), 78
Kidney, hypertension and, 71
Korean War, heart disease during, 9, 10
Kuhlman, W., 76
Kuller, Lewis, 14

Lasagna, 165–66
Leighninger, David, 79
Life expectancies, 14–16
Linoleic acid, 142
Lipemia, 93
Low Cholesterol Diet Manual (Department of Internal Medicine, University of Iowa), 210n
Low-fat diet, diabetes and, 38, 55–59
Low fat/low cholesterol diet, 24–26, 30, 36–37, 41–43
Luyken, R., 53

Macleod, J. J. R., 49
Malaria, 4
Manicotti, 165–66
Mann, George, 82
Masai people (Kenya), hypertension among, 82

Mayer, Jean, 125, 127, 128, 196
Measles, 4
Meats, 146, 151
  browning, 157–58
  cholesterol content of, 211
  composition of, 213–14
Medical profession, 128–29
Menu, sample, 154–55
Merrill, A. L., 213
Mexico City, 1968 Olympics in, 80–81
Minerals, 111–13
Minestrone soup, 163
Minkowski (researcher), 49
Mock Sour Cream, 161
Morrison, L. M., 41–43
Moussaka, 171

National Academy of Sciences, 107, 110
National Heart and Lung Institute, 47
Nedde, William, 82, 83
Neptune Chowder, 169
Netherlands, heart disease in, 11
New Guinea
  fat consumption in, 53–54
  heart disease in, 27
Nicotinic acid, 47
Night blindness, 107
Nkana Nune Hospital, 26
Nonfat dairy products, 146
Nutrition, 86–89
  acceptable food for, 216–18
  alcoholism and, 105
  cholesterol contents of food and, 210–12
  composition of foods and, 212–15
  degenerative diseases and, 141–44
  proteins and, 94–98

Oils, *see* Fats
Orinase, 61–62
Overweight (Mayer), 125, 196
Oxygenation, 79–81

Pancreas
  diabetes and, 49–53
  insulin production by, 59, 60
Papuans (of New Guinea), fat consumption by, 53–54

Pasta, 153
Paul, O., 75
Pellagra, 99
Phenformin, 61–62
Phosphoric acid, 118
Pizza, Venice Combination, 166–67
Plaques, atherosclerosis and, 19, 33–34
Pomeroy, William C., 78
Poultry (chicken), 151
  breading, 158
  cholesterol content of, 211
  recipe for, 170–71
President's Council on Physical Fitness, 77
Priess (researcher), 53, 55
Primitive peoples
  fat consumption by, 53–54
  heart disease among, 25–29
  hypertension among, 82
Probenecid, 72
Proteins (amino acids), 103
  carbohdrates and, 89, 90
  nutrition and, 94–98
Public Health Service, Framingham, Mass., study by, 23, 78

Rabinowitch, I. M., 52, 53
Rainy Day Salad, 160
Reaven, G. M., 51
Recipes, 158–73
  entrees from south of the border, 172–73
  Italian entrees, 165–67
  salads, 159–61
  sea food entrees, 168–69
  soups, 161–64
  specialty entrees, 170–72
Restaurant situation, 203–5
Rickets, 99
Roving, 181–98
  advice on, 187–92
  defined, 181
  exercise program and, 182–85
  physiological benefits of, 18–87
  problem solving and, 194–98
  traveling and, 202–3

Salads, 159–61
  Holiday, 160
  Rainy Day, 160

Salt
  degenerative diseases and, 143
  diet and, 146
  hypertension and, 70, 71
San Francisco, heart disease study in, 24
Santa Barbara Split Pea Soup, 162
Scarlet fever, 4
Schoenberger (researcher), 68
Scurvy, 99
SDA (specific dynamic action), 126–27
Sea food entrees, 168–69
Shephard, Roy, 192n
Shopping list, 148–53
Sleep, 174–75
Small pox, 4
Smoking and Health (U.S. Public Health Service), 73
Society of Actuaries, 65
Soups, 153, 161–64
  Cabbage/Beet Borscht, 164
  Fresh Frozen Pea, 164
  Gazpacho, 162–63
  Green Lentil, 161–62
  Minestrone, 163
  Santa Barbara Split Pea, 162
Spaghetti, 153
  recipe, 165
Spanish Salad Soup (Gazpacho), 162–63
Specialty entrees, 170–72
Stamler, Jeremiah, 140
Starches, 91–93
Stress, 44–46
Stroke, *see* Cerebrovascular disease
Sugar
  carbohydrates and, 55–58
  degenerative disease and, 142–43
  diabetes and, 48
  diet and, 146
  as starch, 91–94
Surgeon General, U.S., 73
Swimming, 194

Taylor, H. L., 78
Tea, caffeine and, 75–76, 143, 145
Thiazides, 72
"350 calorie Pilot's diet," 126
Traveling, 202–3

Triparanol, 46
Tuberculosis, 3–5
Tucker, C., 37
2100 Program
  exercise program of, 178–98
  food program of, 140–77
  helpful hints for, 199–210
  longer life and, 137–38
Typhoid fever, 4

Ulcers, emotional stress and, 44–46
Unidentified essential chemicals, 114–15
United States
  changing disease patterns in, 3–16
  cigarette smoking in, 73
  fat consumption in, 24
University Group Diabetes Program (UGDP), 61–62
Unsaturated fats, 37–44

Veal, 158
Vegetables, 146, 152, 214
  sauteing without fat, 157
Venice Combination Pizza, 166–67
Vietnam War, heart disease during, 9, 10
Vitamins, 98–110
  deficiency symptoms for, 104–6
Von Mering (researcher), 49

Watt, B. K., 213
Weight
  fad diets and, 122–27
  roving and, 196–97
  2100 Program and, 175–76
Weight Watchers, 124
Whooping cough, 4
White, Paul Dudley, 78, 140, 196
Whyte, H. M., 27
Williams, Roger, 105, 106
Wolf (researcher), 53, 55
World Health Organization (WHO), 8

Yalow, R. S., 51
Yugoslavia, heart disease in, 11

NUTRIENTS IN THE EDIBLE PORTION OF 1 POUND OF FOOD AS PURCHASED [3]

Food and description	Refuse (Percent)	Food energy (Calories)	Protein (Grams)	Fat (Grams)	Carbohydrate total (Grams)
APPLES:					
Raw, commercial varieties:[5]					
Freshly harvested and stored, portion used—					
Fruit with skin:					
Good quality (refuse: core, stem)	8	242	.8	2.5	60.5
Fair quality (refuse: core, stem, defects)	18	216	.7	2.2	53.9
Pared fruit:					
Good quality (refuse: core, stem, thin parings)	14	211	.8	1.2	55.0
Fair quality (refuse: core, stems, thin parings, defects)	24	186	.7	1.0	48.6
Freshly harvested, portion used—					
Fruit with skin (refuse: core, stem)	8	234	.8	2.5	58.8
Pared fruit (refuse: core, stem, thin parings)	14	207	.8	1.2	54.2
Stored, portion used—					
Fruit with skin (refuse: core, stem)	8	250	.8	2.9	61.8
Pared fruit (refuse: core, stem, thin parings)	14	215	.8	1.2	56.2
APPLE JUICE: canned or bottled	0	213	.5	.1	54.0
APPLESAUCE, canned:					
Unsweetened or artificially sweetened	0	186	.9	.9	49.0
APRICOTS:					
Raw (12 per lb.) (refuse: pits)	6	217	4.3	.9	54.6
ASPARAGUS:					
Raw spears (refuse: butt ends)	44	66	6.4	.5	12.7
Canned spears:					
Green, solids and liquid:					
Regular pack	0	82	8.6	1.4	13.2
Special dietary pack (low-sodium)	0	73	9.1	.9	12.2
White (bleached) solids and liquid:					
Regular pack	0	82	7.3	1.4	15.0
Special dietary pack (low-sodium)	0	73	6.4	.9	13.6
Frozen:					
Cuts and tips	0	104	15.0	.9	16.3
Spears	0	109	15.0	.9	17.7
BANANAS:					
Raw:					
Common:					
Good quality (refuse: skin)	32	262	3.4	.6	68.5
Fair quality (refuse: skin, defects)	45	212	2.7	.5	55.4

Food and description	Refuse (Percent)	Food energy (Calories)	Protein (Grams)	Fat (Grams)	Carbohydrate total (Grams)
BANANAS: (cont.)					
Red (refuse: skin)	(32)	278	3.7	.6	72.2
Dehydrated, or banana powder (3.0% moisture)	0	1,542	20.0	3.6	401.9
BARLEY, pearled:					
Light	0	1,583	37.2	4.5	357.4
Pot or Scotch	0	1,579	43.5	5.0	350.2
BEANS, COMMON, mature seeds, dry:					
White:					
Raw	0	1,542	101.2	7.3	278.1
Canned, solids and liquid:					
With pork and tomato sauce	0	553	27.7	11.8	86.2
With pork and sweet sauce	0	680	28.1	21.3	95.7
Without pork	0	544	28.6	2.3	104.3
Red:					
Raw	0	1,556	102.1	6.8	280.8
Canned, solids and liquid	0	408	25.9	1.8	74.4
Pinto, calico, and red Mexican, raw	0	1,583	103.9	5.4	288.9
Other, including black, brown, and Bayo, raw	0	1,538	101.2	6.8	277.6
BEANS, LIMA:					
Immature seeds:					
Raw:					
In pod (refuse: pods)	60	223	15.2	.9	40.1
Shelled	0	558	38.1	2.3	100.2
Canned, solids and liquid:					
Regular pack	0	322	18.6	1.4	60.8
Special dietary pack (low-sodium)	0	318	20.0	1.4	58.5
Frozen:					
Thick-seeded types, commonly called Ford-hooks	0	463	28.1	.5	88.5
Thin-seeded types, commonly called baby limas	0	553	34.5	.9	104.3
Mature seeds, dry, raw	0	1,565	92.5	7.3	290.3
BEAN FLOUR, LIMA	0	1,556	97.5	6.4	285.8
BEANS, MUNG, raw:					
Mature seeds, dry	0	1,542	109.8	5.9	273.5
Bean Sprouts	0	159	17.2	.9	29.9
BEEF:					
T-bone steak:					
Choice grade:					
Total edible, with bone, 55% lean, 34% fat	11	1,596	59.1	149.1	0

[1] Estimated average based on addition of salt in the amount of .6% finished product.

[2] Average weighted in accordance with commercial practices in freezing vegetables.

[Numbers in parentheses denote value imputed—usually from another form of the food or from a similar food. Zero in parentheses indicates that the amount of a constituent probably is none or is too small to measure. Question marks denote lack of reliable data for a constituent believed to be present in measurable amount. Calculated values, as those based on recipe, are not in parentheses]

Calcium (Milligrams)	Phosphorus (Milligrams)	Iron (Milligrams)	Sodium (Milligrams)	Potassium (Milligrams)	Vitamin A value (International Units)	Thiamine (Milligrams)	Riboflavin (Milligrams)	Niacin (Milligrams)	Ascorbic acid (Milligrams)
29	42	1.3	4	459	380	.12	.08	.3	16
26	37	1.1	4	409	330	.10	.07	.3	14
23	39	1.2	4	429	160	.11	.07	.3	9
21	34	1.0	3	379	140	.10	.07	.2	8
29	42	1.3	4	459	380	.12	.08	.3	29
23	39	1.2	4	429	160	.11	.07	.3	15
29	42	1.3	4	459	380	.12	.08	.3	14
23	39	1.2	4	429	160	.11	.07	.3	8
27	41	2.7	5	458	?	.03	.07	.4	4
18	23	2.3	9	354	180	.08	.05	.2	5
72	98	2.1	4	1,198	11,510	.14	.16	2.6	.42
56	157	2.5	5	706	2,290	.46	.51	3.9	84
82	195	7.7	1,070[1]	753	2,310	.29	.42	3.7	68
82	195	7.7	14	753	2,310	.29	.42	3.7	68
68	150	4.1	1,070[1]	635	230	.23	.26	3.2	68
68	150	4.1	18	635	230	.23	.26	3.2	68
104	299	5.9	9	1,084	3,860	.73	.64	5.3	114
104	313	5.4	9	1,175	3,540	.82	.68	5.7	132
25	80	2.2	3	1,141	590	.14	.18	2.2	31
20	65	1.7	2	923	470	.12	.15	1.7	25

Calcium (Milligrams)	Phosphorus (Milligrams)	Iron (Milligrams)	Sodium (Milligrams)	Potassium (Milligrams)	Vitamin A value (International Units)	Thiamine (Milligrams)	Riboflavin (Milligrams)	Niacin (Milligrams)	Ascorbic acid (Milligrams)
31	56	2.5	3	1,141	1,230	.15	.12	1.8	(31)
145	472	12.7	18	6,700	3,450	.82	1.07	12.7	29
73	857	9.1	14	726	(0)	.55	.23	14.1	(0)
154	1,315	12.2	?	1,343	(0)	.95	.32	16.8	(0)
653	1,928	35.4	86	5,425	0	2.96	1.02	10.8	?
245	417	8.2	2,100	953	590	.34	.14	2.6	9
286	517	10.4	1,724	?	?	.26	.20	2.3	?
308	549	9.1	1,533	1,216	270	.32	.16	2.5	9
499	1,842	31.3	45	4,463	90	2.33	.92	10.6	?
132	494	8.2	14	1,198	Trace	.23	.18	2.7	?
612	2,073	29.0	45	4,463	?	3.80	.95	10.0	?
612	1,905	35.8	113	4,708	140	2.51	.91	9.8	?
94	528	5.1	4	1,179	530	4.3	.22	2.5	52
236	644	12.7	9	2,948	1,320	1.08	.55	6.4	130
118	304	10.9	1,070[1]	1,007	590	.16	.20	2.4	32
118	304	10.9	18	1,007	590	.16	.20	2.4	32
104	435	8.6	585[2]	2,223	1,040	.45	.27	5.4	101
172	594	12.7	667[2]	1,987	1,000	.45	.27	5.6	85
327	1,746	35.4	18	6,936	Trace	2.17	.75	8.6	?
?	?	?	?	?	(0)	?	?	?	(0)
535	1,542	34.9	27	4,663	360	1.71	.96	11.7	?
86	290	5.9	23	1,012	90	.60	.61	3.4	86
32	543	8.8	250	1,370	300	.25	.53	14.2	?

A COMPLETE HANDBOOK ON THE NUTRIENTS IN FOODS CAN BE OBTAINED BY SENDING $5.00 TO COMPOSITION OF FOODS, P.O. BOX 17873, TUCSON, ARIZONA 85731. THIS 190-PAGE HANDBOOK SHOULD BE OBTAINED BY EVERY PERSON INTERESTED IN HIS GOOD HEALTH AND EVERY PERSON BEGINNING THE 2100 FOOD PROGRAM. IT IS A POWERFUL SUPPLEMENT TO THIS BOOK.

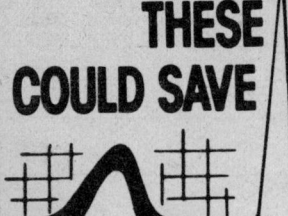

THESE BOOKS COULD SAVE YOUR LIFE!

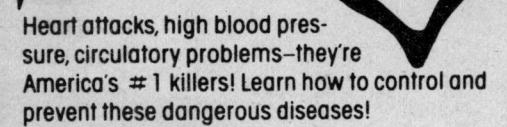

Heart attacks, high blood pressure, circulatory problems—they're America's #1 killers! Learn how to control and prevent these dangerous diseases!

___ 08825-0	**CORONARIES, CHOLESTEROL AND CHLORINE** by J.M. Price	$2.95
___ 08235-X	**RAW VEGETABLE JUICES** by Dr. N.W. Walker	$2.95
___ 08447-6	**THE EDGAR CAYCE HANDBOOK FOR HEALTH** by Dr. Harold J. Reilly and Ruth Hagy Brod	$3.95
___ 08724-6	**ACT THIN, STAY THIN** by Richard B. Stuart	$3.95

Prices may be slightly higher in Canada.

Available at your local bookstore or return this form to:

JOVE
THE BERKLEY PUBLISHING GROUP, Dept. B
390 Murray Hill Parkway, East Rutherford, NJ 07073

Please send me the titles checked above. I enclose _____ Include $1.00 for postage and handling if one book is ordered; 25¢ per book for two or more not to exceed $1.75. California, Illinois, New Jersey and Tennessee residents please add sales tax. Prices subject to change without notice and may be higher in Canada.

NAME_____

ADDRESS_____

CITY_____STATE/ZIP_____

(Allow six weeks for delivery.)

SK29